Guidelines on the Termination of Life-Sustaining Treatment and the Care of the Dying

Medical Ethics series
David H. Smith and Robert M. Veatch, editors

Table of Contents

PREFACE

This document offers comprehensive ethical guidelines for decisions on whether to forgo life-sustaining medical treatment. It concerns the treatment of all patients (except those in infancy*) whose care raises questions about the use of life-sustaining treatment.** Thus, the Guidelines address not only the care of patients known to be dying or terminally ill (as used in these Guidelines, "terminally ill" means likely to die within one year with or without treatment), but also the care of patients who are critically or seriously ill or simply facing a decision about the use of a life-sustaining treatment. Building on previously developed policies and guidelines, these Guidelines represent the culmination of an extensive study by a Hastings Center research group drawn from the fields of medicine, nursing, law, philosophy, and health care administration.

The purpose of the Guidelines is to provide guidance to all concerned with the use of life-sustaining treatment and the care of the seriously ill—physicians, nurses, other health professionals, patients, family members, surrogates, administrators, ethics committees, scholars, and public officials. Probably few patients and family members will consult this document directly, however. Indeed, patients and their families are often the least aware of the ethical responsibilities others owe to them, and that fact increases the burden on those others to act in an ethically responsible way.

These Guidelines are not, however, meant to be hastily consulted by the pressured physician or nurse. They are not the ethical equivalent of a pocket manual offering quick and easy answers at the patient's bedside or in a crisis. The Guidelines ideally should instead be read in their entirety in circumstances that permit reflection and discussion. The individual health care professional will—we hope—find here useful and thought-provoking ethical guidance.

Administrators, ethics committees, and policy makers may find the document to be a helpful basis for formulating policy. Some institutions may conclude that the Guidelines or portions of them should become institutional policy with little change in the basic recommendations. Other institutions may find the Guidelines to be a useful starting point for discussion in developing a somewhat different policy. No single set of guidelines or policy can serve all health care institutions and settings. These Guidelines, moreover, cover some of the most controversial issues in medical ethics. This document is not meant to foreclose but to prompt debate.

These Guidelines are also not intended to substitute for the scholarly literature and reports on forgoing life-sustaining treatment. Our purpose was to distill that work and use it as a starting point in formulating practical guidelines, presenting both concrete recommendations and the rationale behind them. We strongly encourage readers of these Guidelines to consult the literature and explore the debates more deeply; the BIBLIOGRAPHY suggests useful and provocative sources.

The advances of medicine are among the most notable human achievements of the twentieth century. Less than fifty years ago, there were relatively few serious illnesses that health care professionals could effectively treat, let alone cure. Physicians and nurses often could provide only care and comfort, and were unable to alter the natural processes of healing or degeneration. This has dramatically changed. With the development of powerful diagnostic procedures and therapeutic interventions, effective drugs, useful preventive measures, and sophisticated surgical techniques, medical science has eliminated some of the traditional causes of early death, and helped to prolong the average life span. Clearly these advances have brought tremendous human benefit, and we should seek further improvement in medicine's life-saving and life-enhancing capacities.

---

*The care of patients in infancy may raise some unique ethical, policy, and legal issues; those issues are beyond the scope of this document. However, the statutes and regulations on medical abuse and neglect of those patients (see LIST OF SELECTED LEGAL AUTHORITIES) may apply to some of the patients who are covered by these Guidelines.

**See the GLOSSARY for the definition of this and various other terms used in these Guidelines. Some of the confusion surrounding termination of treatment issues stems from ambiguity in the language used; we include a glossary to attempt to eliminate that ambiguity.

But the new powers of medicine have proved to be a mixed blessing. Our capacity to prolong life in many cases exceeds our capacity to restore health. Many medical treatments can sustain vital functioning without being able to reverse the underlying disease processes that may cause suffering or lead to death. The use of these treatments—cardiopulmonary resuscitation, mechanical ventilation, dialysis, feeding tubes, and the like—increasingly poses perplexing ethical and legal dilemmas.

As fewer people experience a quick and unexpected death, more undergo a protracted dying process, often with intensive and invasive medical treatment. Many of these patients find themselves dependent upon life-sustaining treatments and face the prospect of prolonged, expensive, and burdensome care. Patients may not be capable of making decisions about their own treatment, and even patients who have decisionmaking capacity often find it difficult to cope with their problems and to make their own choices. These situations pose difficulties for health care professionals, who must assist with decisionmaking and provide ongoing care.

The guiding philosophy of our health care institutions should be that the health and well-being of the individual patient are the paramount considerations. In keeping with this, there is a legitimate moral and legal presumption in favor of preserving life and providing beneficial medical care with the patient's informed consent. Clearly, however, avoiding death should not always be the preeminent goal; not all technologically possible means of prolonging life need be or should be used in every case.

Deciding when to forgo available life-sustaining treatment raises a host of substantive and procedural issues. In recent years these issues have received considerable attention. Numerous states have adopted legislation on the determination of death and on the use of advance directives to specify what care the individual wants to receive and who should make decisions if a patient loses decisionmaking capacity. A number of state courts have ruled on cases involving the termination of treatment and surrogate decisionmaking. Many hospitals have formulated policies on the use of cardiopulmonary resuscitation and have established institutional ethics committees. Governmental commissions, professional associations, religious and other groups, individual physicians and other health care professionals, legal scholars, and ethicists have written on these issues. Public understanding has gradually increased and society has moved toward greater agreement on ethical matters.

These Guidelines build on those sources, drawing on their insight and addressing topics previously neglected, to offer comprehensive ethical guidance on forgoing life-sustaining treatment and caring for the dying.

These Guidelines are new and different from past work in a number of ways:

- They provide an integrated and comprehensive approach to the ethical issues raised by the termination of treatment and care of the dying.

- They present both a basic decisionmaking format and the procedures and problems peculiar to individual treatment modalities.

- They cover "macro" policy issues that transcend the treatment of any one person as well as "micro" issues raised by the treatment of individual patients.

- They speak not only to physicians, but also to the broader health care team, recognizing the particularly significant role of nurses.

- They address a variety of treatment settings—the hospital, nursing home, hospice, and ambulatory care settings—plus different services and units within the hospital setting.

- They consider not only patients with decisionmaking capacity and those without, but also those of unclear or fluctuating capacity.

- They emphasize prospective planning for life-threatening medical conditions.

- They cover some treatments not widely considered before, particularly in a guidelines format, such as antibiotics and palliative care.

The pages that follow list the permanent members of the project group responsible for these Guidelines. This is a consensus document—an individual project member may not agree with every word, but each subscribes to the document as a whole except as noted in the Dissents. (See APPENDIX.) The Guidelines were drafted largely by the project staff. I would like to thank my colleagues Cynthia Cohen, Bruce Jennings, Paul Homer, and Daniel Callahan for their assistance.

Also listed on the following pages are those who, while not project members, attended our meetings or corresponded with us, and provided criticism and suggestions. Their insights and reactions have proved invaluable. None of them is to be held responsible for the content of these Guidelines.

In addition to these Guidelines, the Project on the Termination of Treatment has produced a collection of cases. The collection is entitled *Casebook on the Termination of Life-Sustaining Treatment and Care of the Dying*, edited by Cynthia B. Cohen. It presents 26 cases, with commentaries written by project members and staff. Each case concerns some problem addressed by the Guidelines and the cases are organized by the major sections of the Guidelines. The collection is an educational resource that can be used either with or without the Guidelines in a wide range of teaching contexts, including medical school, nursing school, residency programs, and continuing education.

We would like to thank Mrs. Shirley S. Katzenbach for the generous support that allowed us to conduct this project and produce the Guidelines and collection of cases. Her interest and loyalty to the project have been unflagging. We would also like to thank the Greenwall Foundation for continuing support of our work in this area.

Finally, the project owes a great debt of thanks to Janet Bower, who tirelessly typed and retyped this manuscript, and handled effectively a great array of administrative chores. Her assistance was superb.

Susan M. Wolf
Project Director

CONTRIBUTORS

TO THE TERMINATION OF TREATMENT GUIDELINES PROJECT*

MEMBERS OF THE HASTINGS CENTER PROJECT ON THE TERMINATION OF TREATMENT AND CARE OF THE DYING

Those in this category are responsible for the Guidelines that follow.

PROJECT DIRECTOR

Susan M. Wolf, J.D.
Associate for Law
The Hastings Center

ASSOCIATE PROJECT DIRECTORS

Cynthia B. Cohen, Ph.D., J.D.
Philosophy Department
Villanova University
formerly Associate for Ethical Studies
The Hastings Center

Bruce Jennings, M.A.
Associate for Policy Studies
The Hastings Center

Paul Homer, M.A.
Assistant to the Director
The Hastings Center

Daniel Callahan, Ph.D.
Director
The Hastings Center

PROJECT STAFF

Janet M. Bower
Administrative Assistant
The Hastings Center

PROJECT MEMBERS

Dan W. Brock, Ph.D.
Professor of Philosophy and Program in Medicine
Brown University

Daniel Callahan, P.h.D.
Director
The Hastings Center

Michael C. Cantor, M.D.
Fellow, Division of Digestive Diseases
New York Hospital/Cornell Medical Center

Eric J. Cassell, M.D.
Clinical Professor of Public Health
Cornell University Medical College

Cynthia B. Cohen, Ph.D., J.D.
Philosophy Department
Villanova University
formerly Associate for Ethical Studies
The Hastings Center

Ronald E. Cranford, M.D.
Associate Physician in Neurology
Hennepin County Medical Center
Minneapolis, MN

Harold Edgar, LL.B.
Julius Silver Professor of Law, Science &
    Technology
Columbia University School of Law

Lois K. Evans, D.N.Sc., R.N.
Assistant Professor
University of Pennsylvania School of Nursing

Paul Homer, M.A.
Assistant to the Director
The Hastings Center

Bruce Jennings, M.A.
Associate for Policy Studies
The Hastings Center

Joanne Lynn, M.D.
Associate Professor
George Washington University Medical Center

Mathy Mezey, Ed.D., R.N.
Professor of Gerontological Nursing and
Director, The Robert Wood Johnson Foundation
    Teaching Nursing Home Program
University of Pennsylvania School of Nursing

---

*Institutional affiliation for identification only.

David H. Miller, M.D.
Director, Coronary Care Unit and
Assistant Professor of Medicine
New York Hospital/Cornell Medical Center

Harry R. Moody, Ph.D.
Deputy Director
Brookdale Center on Aging of Hunter College

Ellen Olson, M.D.
Medical Director
Village Nursing Home
New York City

Ruth Oratz, M.D.
Division of Oncology
Bellevue Hospital
New York University Medical Center

Nicholas Rango, M.D.
Executive Director
Village Nursing Home
New York City

Leslie Steven Rothenberg, J.D.
Clinical Ethicist
Los Angeles, CA

Robert M. Veatch, Ph.D.
Professor of Medical Ethics
Kennedy Institute of Ethics
Georgetown University

Susan M. Wolf, J.D.
Associate for Law
The Hastings Center

ADDITIONAL MEETING PARTICIPANTS

Those in this and the following categories are *not* responsible for the content of the Guidelines.

Mary Ahern
Assistant General Counsel
American Hospital Association

Donna Myers Ambrogi
Directing Attorney
California Law Center on Long Term Care

Susanna E. Bedell
Beth Israel Hospital
Boston, MA

Walter M. Bortz
Health Care Division
Palo Alto Medical Clinic

Tom Bradley
San Francisco VA Medical Center

Cyril Brosnan
President
Health Services Improvement Fund
New York City

Patricia Cahill
Health Care Coordinator
Archdiocese of New York
Providence Health Services
New York City

Courtney Campbell
Associate Editor
Hastings Center Report
The Hastings Center

Patricia Clarke
Staff Member
Office of Honorable James R. Tallon, Jr.
New York State Assembly

Mary A. Cooke
Director, Hospice Program
Cabrini Medical Center
New York City

Ann Alexis Coté
Associate Director
New York Hospital

Mary M. Devlin
Staff Attorney
American Medical Association

Nancy N. Dubler
Director, Division of Legal & Social Medicine
Department of Epidemiology & Social Medicine
Montefiore Hospital and Medical Center
Bronx, NY

Alice Cotter Feldman
Gerontological Nursing Interagency
    Sharing Group
New York City

Jerry Warren
Assistant Vice President
American Baptist Homes of the West

Robert Weir
Chairman, Religious Studies Department
Oklahoma State University

Jonathan A. Weiss
Director
Legal Services for the Elderly

ADDITIONAL CORRESPONDENTS

Marie R. Baldisseri
Presbyterian-University Hospital of Pittsburgh

James Bopp, Jr.
Brames, Bopp, Haynes & Abel
Terre Haute, IN

Lynn Boyd
Legislative Representative
American Association of Retired Persons

Patty D. Brown
Staff Liaison
Bio-Ethics Committee
American College of Emergency Physicians

Sam P. Giordano
Executive Director
American Association for Respiratory Therapy

Ake Grenvik
Professor of Anesthesiology and Surgery
University of Pittsburgh, School of Medicine
Presbyterian-University Hospital

C. Rollins Hanlon
Director
American College of Surgeons

George D. Hanzel
Chest Diseases Ltd
Johnstown, PA

Herbert D. Hinkle
Director
Department of the Public Advocate
Division of Advocacy for the Developmentally
   Disabled
State of New Jersey

Andrew Jameton
Department of Medical Jurisprudence and
   Humanities
University of Nebraska

Joanne Ingalls McKay
Associate Executive Director
Professional Services
Emergency Nurses Association

Charles E. Millard
Chairman
Committee on Medical Ethics
The American Academy of Family Physicians

Jerome H. Modell
Professor and Chairman
Department of Anesthesiology
University of Florida-College of Medicine
Gainesville, FL

Michael A. Nevins
Governor, New Jersey Chapter
American College of Physicians

Roger J. Purdy
Committee on Evolving Trends in Society Affect-
   ing Life
California Medical Association

Gary A. Ratkin
Chairman
Clinical Practice Committee
American Society of Clinical Oncology

Mark R. Reiner
President
North American Transplant Coordinators
   Organization

Colin C. Rorrie, Jr.
Executive Director
American College of Emergency Physicians

Phyllis Rubenfeld
President
American Coalition of Citizens with Disabilities,
  Inc.

Michael Salcman
Secretary
Congress of Neurological Surgeons

Robert L. Sassone
Attorney at Law
Santa Ana, CA

Elaine Shelton
Director
Medical and Scientific Advisory Board Services
Alzheimer's Disease and Related Disorders
  Association, Inc.

Kent Smith
Executive Director
Spina Bifida Association of America

Ann W. Tourigny
Director
Professional Affairs
American College of Health Care Administrators

Carl P. Wiezalis
Program Director, Respiratory Therapy Programs
SUNY Upstate Medical Center
Syracuse, NY

The Organization of the Guidelines

This document is divided into six Parts. PART ONE presents a basic process for ethical decisionmaking on the termination of treatment, then PART TWO contains additional Guidelines on specific treatment modalities. PART TWO builds on PART ONE: The Guidelines on individual treatment modalities in PART TWO state the adjustments to that basic process in PART ONE that are necessary in order to make a decision on the particular treatment in question. Thus, each Section in PART TWO must be read together with PART ONE. PART THREE offers Guidelines on prospective planning about the patient's care and the use of life-sustaining treatments, particularly planning by means of formal advance directives. PART FOUR sets forth Guidelines on the determination of death. PART FIVE takes up three sets of policy considerations: institutional ethics committees, institutional policies on patient admissions and transfers, and the role of economic considerations in decisions concerning life-sustaining treatment. PART SIX presents an expanded discussion of certain key problems. The Guidelines include a GLOSSARY, a selected BIBLIOGRAPHY divided by topic, a LIST OF SELECTED LEGAL AUTHORITIES with the citations of important cases and other authorities relevant to the termination of treatment, and an INDEX. An APPENDIX contains two dissents.

INTRODUCTION

I. The Status of the Guidelines and the Role of Law

II. The Scope of the Guidelines

III. The Ethical Framework

IV. The Clinical Context

V. The Importance of Prospective Planning

VI. Basic Goals of Institutional Policy

INTRODUCTION

For the gravely ill patient, and for his or her family, friends, and health care professionals, decisions about the use of life-sustaining treatment have profound consequences. These decisions will, to some extent, hasten or forestall the time of death. And they will shape the patient's experience of remaining life—where it is lived, with whom, and with what comfort or suffering.

These decisions also have an inevitable social dimension. The specific decisions and the decisionmaking process have social, economic, and moral consequences that affect our society as a whole. They compel us, as a society, to examine our ethical priorities— our respect for life, our respect for individual autonomy and dignity, and our understanding of the ultimate goals of medicine. They confront us with issues of justice, equity, and the economic constraints on the use of scarce medical resources.

Even at the bedside, societal factors impinge upon decisions. For patients and health care professionals alike, choice is constrained by prior institutional decisions, by laws, and by public policy choices—all of which limit the available options and medical resources. Nor do these decisions take place in a cultural vacuum. Even the most intimate ethical decisions necessarily reflect the diverse ethical and religious values in our society.

Choices about whether to use or forgo life-sustaining treatment ideally should be informed by ethical values, principles, and analysis that have withstood the test of public scrutiny and debate. Our society must be confident that the decisionmaking process is equitable in the claims it allows individuals to make on health care resources, and just in the protection it affords to the most vulnerable among us. Patients, health care professionals, and others who face these issues must be able to base their decisions on well-founded ethical principles and moral norms.

The purpose of the *Guidelines on the Termination of Life-Sustaining Treatment and the Care of the Dying* is to set forth an integrated, comprehensive framework of ethical guidelines to respond to this need.

I. The Status of these Guidelines and the Role of Law

The ethical Guidelines in this document are intended to provide guidance on the use of life-sustaining treatments. They do not provide an infallible formula for making correct decisions. They are not the ethical version of "cookbook medicine." Their purpose is to guide moral reflection and judgment; they do not eliminate the need to exercise these faculties.

No set of guidelines can or should eliminate the need to respect each patient's unique values and needs; treatment decisions must be made on a case-by-case basis after carefully assessing the benefits and burdens that health care options entail. Nonetheless, guidelines can provide a framework to structure decisionmaking and to ensure consideration of the relevant facts and values. Guidelines can clarify the rights and responsibilities of each participant in the decisionmaking process. Guidelines can help to reassure society that these important decisions are made with proper deliberation and accountability.

These ethical Guidelines have a normative rather than a legal status. They are intended to clarify what conduct is ethically prohibited, ethically permissible, and ethically required; they also set forth positive ideals. Although they contain recommendations that may be incorporated into statutes, judicial decisions, administrative rules, or institutional policies, the Guidelines themselves have no legally binding authority. Their claim to serious attention and their moral force will spring from the informed and reasoned ethical positions they present and from the widely acknowledged standards of ethically responsible medical practice they incorporate.

In formulating these Guidelines, we have been attentive to the state of the law. However, these Guidelines are no substitute for legal advice and users of this document should find out how the law in their jurisdiction bears on the recommendations.

Although these Guidelines differ from law in their status and authority, they are related to the law. The Guidelines, particularly those on decisionmaking procedures, can help policymakers, legislators, and judges identify where more explicit legal direction is needed and where existing law impedes ethical decisionmaking, either directly or by creating uncertainty. The ethical Guidelines offered here may also provide model formulations that, if translated appropriately, can be incorporated into the language of statutes, administrative regulations, and judicial rulings. However, that requires lawmakers to decide which of our ethical recommendations should become law; not all ethical standards should be so converted.

Health care professionals have become increasingly concerned about lawsuits and even about the possibility of criminal prosecution. Although the law serves a legitimate function in setting limits to behavior, it would be a mistake to allow medical care to become shaped primarily by legal concerns. The primary concern should be the patient's welfare. Hospital legal counsel, lawyers serving other health care institutions, and legal advisors to individual health care professionals have a critical role to play in seeing that medicine is not driven by law, and health care professionals are not preoccupied by legal concerns. These lawyers need to educate themselves fully on the law concerning the termination of treatment. They then must educate health care professionals about the law, eliminating the misinformation that is now rampant, and creating an atmosphere in which health care professionals can practice medicine without also trying to practice law.

Since the landmark *Quinlan* case in 1976, many courts have recognized the patient's right to forgo life-sustaining treatment. (See LIST OF SELECTED LEGAL AUTHORITIES.) Although the courts vary in the procedures they recommend, including whether recourse to the courts is necessary, generally cases of forgoing treatment need not routinely go to court. Some states have passed statutes that establish procedures for forgoing life-sustaining treatment. The California "Natural Death Act" is an example. (See LIST OF SELECTED LEGAL AUTHORITIES.) That statute, among other things, recognizes the propriety of advance directives—directions that the patient gives to health care professionals while he or she still has decisionmaking capacity, stating what course of treatment the patient wants should he or she later lack capacity. More and more states are enacting legislation that allows people to make advance directives.

Built-in features of the law should also reassure health care professionals. The law on forgoing life-sustaining treatment is not developing in isolation from ethics or public sentiment. Many judicial decisions in the area cite and discuss ethics authorities, and the public consensus that is developing on these issues undoubtedly affects prosecutors considering whether to bring a criminal proceeding, as well as legislators and judges. Furthermore, as of this date there has been no successful criminal prosecution for the withdrawal of life-sustaining treatment.

II. The Scope of the Guidelines

Life-sustaining treatment is any medical intervention, technology, procedure, or medication that is administered to a patient in order to forestall the moment of death, whether or not the treatment is intended to affect the underlying life-threatening disease(s) or biologic processes. Examples include ventilators, dialysis, and cardiopulmonary resuscitation.

Questions about forgoing life-sustaining treatment will ordinarily arise when death is the predictable or unavoidable outcome of the patient's underlying medical condition. However, a patient need not be terminally ill or imminently dying for these decisions to be ethically permissible. Hence these Guidelines cover a broad class of gravely impaired or critically ill patients and others who are not necessarily in danger of imminent death, but who are facing a decision about the use of a life-sustaining treatment.

Similarly, the Guidelines encompass a wide range of medical treatments, including those sometimes classified as "ordinary" and those sometimes labeled "extraordinary." The terms "extraordinary" and "ordinary" are often used in an attempt to distinguish a class of treatments that may ethically be withheld or withdrawn from a class of treatments that may not. We have found that these terms obscure ethically important questions rather than helping to resolve them.

People sometimes distinguish "ordinary" from "extraordinary" treatment by appealing to the prevalence of a treatment or its level of technological complexity. This is misleading because it focuses attention on factors that are ethically irrelevant to the decision to forgo treatment. Certain procedures for providing artificial nutrition and hydration, for example, are technologically rather complex, while administering chemotherapy is not; but it clearly does not follow that the latter is ethically required because it is "ordinary" (technically simple) while the former is optional because it is "extraordinary" (technically complex).

We reject the distinction. No treatment is intrinsically "ordinary" or "extraordinary." All treatments that impose undue burdens on the patient without overriding benefits or that simply provide no benefits may justifiably be withheld or withdrawn. While traditional definitions of "extraordinary" hinged on this comparison of benefits and burdens, the term has become so confusing that it is no longer useful.

These Guidelines encompass both decisions to withhold life-sustaining treatment and decisions to withdraw such treatment once it has begun. Our choice of the phrase "termination of treatment" should not be construed to suggest that the Guidelines refer only to withdrawal of treatment. That is not the case. A decision not to initiate a treatment and a decision to stop a treatment are both subject to ethical analysis; both may be ethically justifiable, depending upon the circumstances.

Many health care professionals and others seem to believe that withholding life-sustaining treatment may be morally permissible, but that withdrawing treatment is wrong. This categorical distinction between withholding and withdrawing treatment seems to us mistaken. There certainly are psychological differences between withholding and withdrawing treatment. But these differences are only the starting point of ethical reflection; they do not determine its conclusions. It is sometimes psychologically more difficult to withdraw treatment than to withhold it, for withdrawal may be perceived as violating a special commitment the health care professional has made to the patient. However, it is usually better to initiate a treatment provisionally, with a plan for stopping it if it proves ineffective or unduly burdensome to the patient, than to withhold a treatment altogether for fear that stopping will be impossible. Indeed, a professional who withholds a treatment without even trying it may be denying the patient a treatment that may prove beneficial. (See also PART SIX: Section II.)

Finally, under the rubric of "termination of treatment," we do not include active euthanasia ("mercy killing") or assisted suicide. These Guidelines have been formulated in the belief that a reasonable, if not unambiguous, line can be drawn between forgoing life-sustaining treatment on the one hand, and active euthanasia or assisted suicide on the other.

Our society forbids assisting suicide or active euthanasia, even if the motive is compassionate. This prohibition serves to sustain the societal value of respect for life and to provide some safeguards against abuse of the authority to take actions that shorten life. It also encourages us to provide decent and humane care to those who suffer, and to those who are dependent, ill, or impaired. Since these people are already vulnerable to being mistreated, undertreated, or avoided, eroding the legal prohibition of active euthanasia might well further endanger them. Respecting the individual's liberty to direct his or her own life requires, however, that patients generally be allowed to refuse medical interventions, even if others feel that this is contrary to the patient's best interests. Likewise, when a person is suffering greatly, medication and other medical interventions may be used to give relief. This relief may foreseeably lead to an earlier death. Yet it may still be morally and legally acceptable, if the intention is not to kill but to relieve the suffering, if the intervention proposed serves the patient's needs better than would any alternative, and if the patient or surrogate consents. We discuss the problem further in PART SIX: Section I.

III. The Ethical Framework

The ethical values that inform the Guidelines come from the

moral traditions of medicine and nursing and from the ethical, religious, and legal traditions of our society. We have identified four central values. All are important and the order in which we discuss them is not meant to rank their relative significance.

The first key value is the patient's well-being. A long tradition of medical ethics acknowledges that the proper goal of medicine is to promote the patient's well-being. In medical ethics this is often called the principle of beneficence.

Second, our ethical framework draws on the value of patient autonomy or self-determination, which establishes the right of the patient to determine the nature of his or her own medical care. This value reflects our society's long-standing tradition of recognizing the unique worth of the individual. We respect human dignity by granting individuals the freedom to make choices in accordance with their own values. The principle of autonomy is the moral basis for the legal doctrine of informed consent, which includes the right of informed refusal.

In applying the value of autonomy to decisions to forgo life-sustaining treatment, we place the patient at the center of the decisionmaking process. Respecting autonomy means that patients with decisionmaking capacity have the right to make these decisions. A patient has decisionmaking capacity* when the patient has (a) the ability to comprehend information relevant to the decision at hand, (b) the ability to deliberate in accordance with his or her own values and goals, and (c) the ability to communicate with caregivers. Except in emergency situations where the patient's prior determination is unknown, medical treatment should not be imposed on a patient with decisionmaking capacity against his or her will or without his or her informed consent. Conversely, life-sustaining treatment that others in similar circumstances routinely receive should not be withheld or withdrawn from a patient with decisionmaking capacity without that patient's informed refusal.

If a patient lacks decisionmaking capacity, respecting autonomy means that an appropriate surrogate (see GLOSSARY) should make

---

*Historically there has been some confusion concerning usage of the terms "competence" and "capacity." Strictly speaking, only the courts have the authority to declare a person "incompetent." Absent a judicial determination, the law presumes competence in adults. Nonetheless, many people refer to the patient who apparently lacks capacity to make treatment decisions as being "incompetent," even when the courts have not been involved in the determination. Technically, such a patient should be referred to as someone who lacks decisionmaking capacity rather than as a person who is "incompetent." Accordingly, the Guidelines use the term "capacity" when referring to a determination outside of court. (See PART SIX: Section III.)

decisions based (a) on the patient's explicit directions, or (b) if there are none, on knowledge of the patient's preferences and values, or (c) if sufficient knowledge is not available, on the basis of how a reasonable person in the patient's circumstances would choose.

A third significant value is the integrity of health care professionals. Physicians, nurses, and other health care professionals have stringent ethical obligations to the patient by virtue of their professional status and role. But they also have a right to remain true to their own conscientious moral and religious beliefs. A system of ethical decisionmaking concerning the use of life-sustaining treatment should be flexible enough to accommodate these beliefs without compromising the legitimate rights of patients and the highest standards of professional care. Thus provisions should be made to allow health care professionals to withdraw from particular cases as a matter of conscience, and for the orderly transfer of the patient to the care of others.

Finally, our framework includes the value of justice or equity. This pertains both to the individual patient's access to an adequate level of health care, and to the distribution of available health care resources. Justice demands that individuals have an opportunity to obtain the health care they need on an equitable basis. At the same time, justice places ethical limits on the patient's liberty to demand, rather than forgo, scarce medical resources. Justice tempers patient autonomy in those cases where complying with the patient's directives would unfairly deprive others of equitable access to an adequate level of scarce medical resources. Considerations of justice or equity enter into decisions concerning the use of life-sustaining treatment (especially at an institutional or policy level) because those treatments can be extremely costly. Providing them can tie up scarce resources (such as beds in the Intensive Care Unit), which must therefore be denied to others.

All of these values play an integral role in medical decisionmaking generally and termination of treatment decisions in particular. We believe that it is proper to place considerable weight on patient autonomy. But neither medical decisionmaking in general nor termination of treatment decisions in particular can be adequately guided by a single value. Each of the above values tempers, and is tempered by, the others. It is not possible to give these principles an absolute rank-ordering. Autonomy, well-being, integrity, and justice must all be given due weight and be woven together into an ethical framework for decisionmaking.

Because decisions about the termination of life-sustaining treatment help determine the timing and circumstances of death, there are also other important social, ethical, and religious values that come into play. Foremost among these is the value commonly referred to as the sanctity of life. This moral value places the burden of proof on those who would foreshorten life or fail to forestall death. In its secular form, the sanctity of life notion draws on the presumption that existence is preferable to non-existence, and that every individual is valuable and unique. In its religious form, it draws on a conviction that life is sacred, and hence individuals may not dispose of it as they choose.

Due regard for the sanctity of life can guard against the erosion of respect for life in our society. By creating a presumption in favor of continued treatment, the sanctity of life can also help to protect gravely ill patients who are vulnerable. This presumption can reassure society that termination of treatment decisions are being made by individuals, institutions, or by society only after careful scrutiny and justification, and not out of ethically illicit motives. Sanctity of life, however, is a presumption; it does not by itself determine whether a particular treatment is appropriate for a patient.

IV. The Clinical Context

Decisions about whether to use or forgo life-sustaining treatment occur in the context of a relationship between health care professional and patient. Discussions of these decisions sometimes present the issues as though health care professionals and patients are adversaries in the process. This is not in any way the perspective of these Guidelines.

The norms of medical practice from their Hippocratic origins have rested on the duty to act in the best interests of the patient. The norms of nursing rest on the same base. Ideally, it is the best interests of the patient as defined by the patient that caregivers must honor. Yet health care professionals may have trouble being guided by what the patient believes to be in his or her best interests for several reasons. Medical knowledge and training for physicians in particular is primarily concerned with the body, but maintaining biological function may not be identical with acting in the best interests of the patient. Technological capacities—especially the ability to support isolated physiologic functions—may create seemingly irresistible imperatives to go ahead and use a treatment; the idea that the patient's interests may not be best served by the treatment may get lost in the few critical minutes when it is most crucial that it be remembered. Illness may also make it hard for the patient to know what he or she thinks best, because of distracting symptoms, fear, denial, unsupported hopes, misconceptions, impairments in thinking, impatience, or conflicting advice. These factors make the task of health care professionals more difficult, but ignoring the patient's definition of his or her own interests will leave the health care professional defining unilaterally what is best for the patient, and will risk making patients and caregivers adversaries at a time when patients most need to trust and believe in their caregivers.

Although illness, especially life-threatening illness, can impede the patient's judgment, only the patient can know what he or she holds to be most important. Finding out what the patient believes to be in his or her best interests may require careful help from the health care professional, allowing the sick person to get beyond the distraction of symptoms, discomfort, and fearfulness. It is this kind of interaction between health care professional and patient that can give reality to the concept of autonomy in dire clinical circumstances.

Caregivers may believe that they do not have the time to engage in such dialogue. However, time spent in discussion with the patient early on may avoid considerable trouble and conflict later. When the patient and caregiver have had a long relationship, it will be less difficult to find out how the patient defines his or her best interests. Often, however, the relationship will not have a long history. In emergency circumstances, it is impossible to have the searching discussions that may be necessary to find out what the patient wants. Because medical emergencies are common, we advocate advance planning throughout these Guidelines. Whenever the patient faces a course of illness in which a termination of treatment decision may arise, the responsible health care professional should begin early exploring the patient's goals and beliefs about termination of treatment. Such discussions are part of the patient's care. They enable the caregiver to supply the information and support needed. Without those discussions, the patient may feel left alone to deal with impossible questions.

When the patient lacks decisionmaking capacity, early discussion and planning with a surrogate is equally necessary. Decisions may be even more difficult for surrogates than for patients themselves. Virtually all close relatives and friends involved in a patient's illness and death feel anxiety and guilt—frequently wondering whether they should do more or act differently. Because of this it is grossly unfair to approach a relative or friend for the first time at 2 a.m. outside an Intensive Care Unit for a decision about the termination of treatment. On occasion, circumstances require an immediate response. Most often, however, the issues can be discussed over a period of time in advance of the moment of action. Then overall goals, rather than an isolated episode, can be discussed with the surrogate. Only in this manner will the patient's or surrogate's choices be integrated into a plan of treatment. The attitude of the caregiver with surrogates, as with patients, should be one of cooperatively seeking what the patient would have wanted.

The most difficult situation is when the patient lacks decisionmaking capacity but has no family or friend to act as a surrogate. This places special burdens on the health care providers, who may have very little information about the patient in order to ascertain what the patient would want. As we recommend in PART ONE, a surrogate should be appointed if at all possible to collaborate with the health care providers in deciding whether to terminate treatment.

The possibility of terminating treatment should be discussed in advance among the members of the health care team. Everyone who may be responsible for the patient should be fully aware of the patient's or surrogate's desires. If at all possible, the task of determining the patient's or surrogate's wishes should not fall to a caregiver who does not know the patient, family, or clinical situation beyond the bare facts on the chart.

Respecting the patient's autonomy requires vital clinical skills. Unless health care professionals learn how to find out what patients really want for themselves and learn to translate this into clinical acts, autonomy will remain an empty concept in medical practice.

Throughout these Guidelines the phrase "responsible health care professional" is used to refer to the health care professional with primary responsibility for a patient's care. Typically, this will be a physician. However, in many instances, particularly in nursing homes and in the context of home health care, a nurse (or more rarely, another health care professional) will be the primary caregiver. The decisionmaking process and the ethical values discussed in these Guidelines apply equally to all health care professionals with primary responsibility for a patient's care.

When the responsible health care professional is not a physician, the responsible professional will need to consult with a physician about some aspects of the patient's care. Some matters will require a physician's expertise; there also may be legal restrictions on what a nurse (or other health care professional who is not a physician) can and cannot do, and what tasks require a physician. These Guidelines speak generically of the "responsible health care professional" who has primary responsibility for the patient's care; professionals should check the standards and law that apply to their practice in order to determine the relevant restrictions and requirements.

These Guidelines emphasize the need to identify one health care professional to assume primary responsibility for the patient's care, but many others are almost invariably involved. No member of the health care team should be cut off from the others, particularly when termination of treatment decisions arise. Open and constructive interprofessional relationships can help to ensure that all are able to voice their concerns, and that the patient or surrogate, as well as health care professionals, get whatever support and counsel they need.

V. The Importance of Prospective Planning

A growing number of individuals are thinking ahead to the kind of care they wish to receive at the end of their lives or after they have become incapable of deciding for themselves. Many people are turning to legal instruments such as "living wills" and other advance directives in order to put their preferences on record and to designate a person to act as a surrogate health care decisionmaker. Even when those legal instruments are not used, prospective planning and discussions among individuals, their health care professionals, and other significant advisors—such as family, friends, and clergy—will usually prove helpful.

Planning should begin well before the onset of the pain and suffering of a progressive illness and before the loss of decisionmaking capacity. Beginning a planning process in the ambulatory setting will greatly reduce the uncertainty and difficulty of termination of treatment decisions. It will also give greater substance to the decisions made—they will be more informed and reflect more extended thought.

If the groundwork has been laid by careful planning, decisionmaking within health care institutions becomes significantly easier. Unfortunately, advance planning is presently far more the exception than the rule. Even with advance planning, problems may arise, particularly in decisionmaking about the termination of treatment.

Termination of treatment decisions are made in a variety of institutional settings. These include ambulatory settings, Emergency Rooms, Intensive Care Units, the medical and surgical services of hospitals, nursing homes or other long-term care facilities, and hospices. Attitudes toward life-sustaining treatment naturally differ among these settings. They may be quite different for example, in an Intensive Care Unit than in a nursing home, or in a large metropolitan teaching hospital as opposed to a rural community hospital. This reality of our health care system makes it important to plan ahead about patient transfers between settings.

VI. Basic Goals of Institutional Policy

Too often institutional rules and policies are followed in an empty and ritualistic way, sometimes in the hope of protecting against legal action. These Guidelines should not be read to suggest a whole new set of legalistic rules, but rather to recommend an ethical basis for decisions on life-sustaining treatment.

Some institutions may consider translating part or all of these Guidelines into institutional policy. The text of the Guidelines indicates our recommendations on specific topics. Here it is sufficient to mention basic objectives that the Guidelines envision for institutional policies on life-sustaining treatment.

Institutional policies and procedures should be sufficiently clear and detailed to assign specific responsibilities to various participants in the decisionmaking process. They should also establish a mechanism for resolving disagreement and conflict. Patients should be notified of these policies before they enter the institution, or as soon after admission as possible. Policies should provide for fair decisionmaking for all patients and should assure accountability so that patients, health care professionals, and society at large may be confident that institutional decisions are not arbitrary or ill-informed.

Policies and the people applying them should foster a climate of dialogue and consultation. Patients should not be left to make termination of treatment decisions in isolation. They must be assured that a decision to forgo a particular treatment option will not mean that caregivers abandon them. Clear institutional policies should reassure patients that a decision to forgo a certain form of life-sustaining treatment will not deprive them of other forms of appropriate medical and nursing care.

Policies should promote accurate and timely communication among health care professionals, to allow the professionals to address concerns and problems and correct mistakes. A decision to use or forgo a life-sustaining treatment should be documented in the patient's medical records, with an explanation of the basis for the decision. Clear responsibility should be assigned to a particular person for maintaining these records and ensuring that all health care professionals involved in the case understand what forms of care the patient is to receive under various circumstances.

Finally, institutional policies should be disseminated through educational programs, so that staff members understand the rationale for the policies and the spirit in which they should be implemented. Without the understanding and cooperation of those who carry them out, no policies can realize their objectives.

HOW TO READ PARTS ONE, TWO, & THREE

PART ONE sets out general guidelines for an ethical decisionmaking process about whether to use or forgo a life-sustaining treatment. This process will require adjustment depending on the treatment at issue. Decisions about whether to use cardiopulmonary resuscitation in the event of a cardiac arrest, for instance, will require some different processes and considerations than decisions about medical procedures for supplying nutrition. Individual Sections in PART TWO of this document address how the basic decisionmaking format set forth in PART ONE should be adjusted for a number of different treatment modalities. To decide about ventilator use, for example, the reader should consult PART ONE together with the Section in PART TWO on ventilators. The INDEX to the Guidelines should also help locate the Sections that pertain to a given treatment.

All of the material in PART ONE applies to each Section in PART TWO unless otherwise stated; each Section in PART TWO contains only the amendments or additions to PART ONE recommended when making decisions about that particular treatment. We use two techniques to make clear where those amendments fit into PART ONE. First, we signal in the text of PART ONE wherever there is an amendment in a Section of PART TWO. For instance, (1)(c) of PART ONE is amended by the Guidelines on ventilators, so the phrase "[*See also Ventilators*]" appears under (1)(c) in the text of PART ONE. Second, the numbering in Sections in PART TWO corresponds to the numbering in PART ONE. For example, the Guidelines on antibiotics in PART TWO elaborate on (2) and (4) of PART ONE, but not (3), and are numbered accordingly. In PART TWO, if a Section contains additional material that does not amend PART ONE, that appears at the end of the Section under "Special comments."

PART THREE: Prospective Planning also complements the basic decisionmaking process set forth in PART ONE. PART THREE concerns planning ahead about treatment and the use of advance directives. This Part advocates beginning the planning process as early as possible, so that the decisionmaking process described in PART ONE can build on accurate information, an understanding of the patient's preferences, and trust.

PART ONE:
Making Treatment Decisions
*GUIDELINES ON THE DECISIONMAKING
PROCESS*

I. INTRODUCTION

II. GUIDELINES ON THE DECISIONMAKING
  PROCESS

(1) Underlying ethical values
   (a) Patient well-being—benefiting more than burdening the
       patient
   (b) Patient self-determination
   (c) The ethical integrity of health care professionals
   (d) Justice or equity

(2) Evaluation and discussion
   (a) Evaluating the patient
   (b) Facilitating discussion

(3) Identifying the key decisionmaker
   (a) Assessing decisionmaking capacity
   (b) Identifying a surrogate
   (c) The patient who lacks a ready surrogate

(4) Making the decision
   (a) The patient with decisionmaking capacity
   (b) The patient whose capacity is fluctuating or uncertain
   (c) The patient who lacks decisionmaking capacity

(5) Documenting the decision

(6) Implementing the decision
   (a) Time-limited trials
   (b) Supportive care
   (c) Maximal therapeutic care
   (d) Stress and communication

(7) Changing the decision

(8) Objections and challenges
    (a) Challenging the determination of lack of capacity
    (b) Challenging a surrogate
    (c) Futility
    (d) Disagreement on the health care team
    (e) Withdrawal of health care professional or institution

(9) Special comments
    (a) Children

PART ONE:
Making Treatment Decisions
GUIDELINES ON THE DECISIONMAKING PROCESS

I. INTRODUCTION

This Part sets forth the outlines of an ethical decisionmaking process on whether to use a life-sustaining treatment. It cannot address all the variations in relations between the patient and the responsible health care professional, and cannot capture the full complexity of any one relationship. Some patients and professionals have a long-standing relationship and rapport before they ever confront a decision about forgoing life-sustaining treatment; others are virtual strangers, meeting each other for the first time when the decision must be made. Moreover, some patients are surrounded by attentive family members who play an active role in treatment decisions; others are completely alone. The interactions of all involved and the decisionmaking process will differ depending on these and other factors. It is possible, however, to generalize and make some recommendations about that process despite the great variation.

Many decisions about life-sustaining treatment already tacitly incorporate the recommendations of these Guidelines: The physician or other responsible health care professional and patient, perhaps with involved family members, consult together; the professional offers recommendations and the patient brings to bear his or her values in making decisions; when the patient is unable to make treatment decisions, a natural decisionmaker emerges from the family. In such cases, there is no need to be more formal or use the precise labels in these Guidelines. A need for clarity forces the Guidelines to be more schematic than the process is in real life. These Guidelines counsel a decisionmaking process that incorporates the basic features recommended; it is not meant to be a rigid sequence of steps for all to march through in case after case.

II. GUIDELINES ON THE DECISIONMAKING PROCESS

(1) **Underlying ethical values.** Decisions about the use of life-sustaining treatment call into play several key ethical values. Their order below is not meant to suggest their relative importance.

(a) **Patient well-being — benefiting more than burdening the patient.** The obligation to promote the good of the patient is basic to the relationship between the health care professional and patient. A decision about whether to use life-sustaining treatment raises the question of whether it will promote the patient's good. Extending life is usually, but not always, a good—the patient's life, for example, may be full of pain or suffering and the patient may prefer to forgo the treatment even though it means an earlier death. Individual patients evaluate the benefits and burdens of a treatment and the life it offers differently. Consequently, the obligation to promote the patient's good involves identifying the benefits and burdens of the treatment from the patient's perspective. Then the question becomes: do the burdens of the treatment outweigh its benefits from the patient's perspective? If they do, it is ethically acceptable to withhold or withdraw the treatment. When, however, the treatment provides more benefits than burdens from the patient's perspective, treatment should be provided. When it is unclear whether the burdens or benefits are greater, it is appropriate to err on the side of life and provide the treatment. If a treatment is clearly futile in the sense that it will not achieve its physiological objective and so offers no physiological benefit to the patient, there is no obligation to provide the treatment. However, such treatment may be provided, particularly when it offers psychological benefit. (See Section (8) (c), p. 32.)
[*See also* **Antibiotics,** *p. 66;* **Palliative Care,** *p. 73*]

(b) **Patient self-determination.** Patients have a right to make important decisions about the course of their life for themselves. One aspect of this right is patients' right to control what happens to their bodies, which implies that the decision about whether to use life-sustaining treatment should in the final analysis be theirs. This is often referred to as the patient's right to self-determination or autonomy. It means that a decision about whether to use life-sustaining treatment requires a decision by the patient who has decisionmaking capacity; for the patient who has no decisionmaking capacity a surrogate decides. But this should happen in the context of a collaborative relationship with health care professionals—indeed, with the professionals' help, support, and counsel.
[*See also* **Bleeding,** *p. 52;* **Palliative Care,** *p. 73*]

(c) **The ethical integrity of health care professionals.** Health care professionals have a clear responsibility to act in accordance with the ethical mandates of their professions and reasonable standards of practice. One of their obligations is to respect the considered choice of the patient or the patient's surrogate and to affirm the values of compassion and human dignity. The health care professional who stops or refrains from using a life-sustaining treatment when the patient or surrogate makes an ethically appropriate decision to forgo it, acts in keeping with the ethical mandates of his or her profession.

Some health care professionals have personal commitments to ethical or religious mandates that raise issues in the course of caring for patients. A health care professional is not required to violate such personal commitments. When the patient or surrogate opts for a course of action that violates the health care professional's personal ethical or religious commitments, the professional should discuss the problem with the patient or surrogate. It may be necessary to transfer the case to another professional with the patient's or surrogate's consent. (See Section (8) (e), p. 32.)
[*See also* **Ventilators**, *p. 39;* **CPR**, *p. 48;* **Palliative Care**, *p. 73*]

(d) Justice or equity. The health care professional's first obligation is to his or her patient. Particularly in an era of cost-cutting and economic pressures, the professional must sometimes struggle to get the services and resources the patient needs. However, in some circumstances the needs of others must impinge on a patient's care. (See PART FIVE: Section C.)
[*See also* **Bleeding**, *p. 52;* **Antibiotics**, *p. 66*]

(2) Evaluation and discussion. It is important that some health care professional be assigned primary responsibility for a patient's care. The health care professional responsible for the patient's care plays a critical role in evaluation and discussion, and in every other aspect of the decisionmaking process as well. If the responsible professional is not a physician, a physician should also be assigned to the patient, and take an active role in the patient's care.

(a) Evaluating the patient. The responsible health care professional must evaluate the patient's current condition as a necessary foundation for any decision about the use of life-sustaining treatment. Sometimes the first person to realize the need for evaluation is not the responsible professional, but another member of the health care team. Those working most closely with the patient are often the first to recognize increasing debilitation, lack of responsiveness to treatment, and other indications of burden to the patient. They also may be the first to realize that the patient, family, or concerned others are considering whether the patient should forgo a treatment. Any member of the health care team should be able to request an evaluation, as should the patient, surrogate, family, or concerned friends. In performing the evaluation, the responsible professional should consult with other members of the health care team, such as physicians, nurses, and social workers. Nurses often have particularly pertinent information, because they provide round-the-clock care.

The responsible professional should not always subject the patient to burdensome testing to reach a diagnosis. Rather the professional should exercise discretion, in consultation with the patient or surrogate, in deciding how much certainty is needed and with what burden as perceived by the patient. There is often diagnostic or prognostic uncertainty when decisions about forgoing treatment must be made. Candor not only about what is known, but also about what is not known, is a part of fully informing the patient or surrogate and laying the groundwork for good decisionmaking. Optimally, an evaluation will yield the following information, with varying degrees of certainty:

1. the patient's diagnosis;

2. the patient's prognosis;

3. the treatment options, their possible benefits and burdens for the patient and the likelihood of each, the effects of each option on the patient's prognosis, and the professional's recommendation;

4. a determination of whether the patient has previously expressed treatment preferences through an advance directive or other means (see PART THREE); and

5. a determination of whether there are family members or concerned others available to participate in the decision-making process.

At all times in the course of care, the responsible health care professional and patient or surrogate should be careful to consider all possible alternative futures that the patient might experience. Often there are more possibilities than are apparent on initial review. When a patient wishes to consider an unconventional course of treatment, the responsible health care professional should collaborate in the decisionmaking process by delineating the nature and length of the future that such treatment might offer.

Reevaluation should be ongoing, with a fuller reevaluation whenever new decisions must be made or the patient's situation changes.

[*See also* **Dialysis,** *p. 41;* **Bleeding,** *p. 52;* **Nutrition,** *p. 60;*
Antibiotics, *p. 66;* **Palliative Care,** *p. 73*]

(b) Facilitating discussion. The evaluation should begin a
process of discussion and interaction—with the patient, and also
with family members or concerned friends, if the patient wants
them involved. Proceeding to a decision about the use of life-
sustaining treatment will involve further discussion—of the
patient's condition, the treatment options, their pros and cons
and potential effects on prognosis, their effect on the patient's
setting, the health care professional's recommendations, and most
importantly the patient's concerns and questions, the patient's
preferences, and how the patient sees the future. This joins the
health care professional's expertise, experience, and concern with
the patient's values and preferences in the decisionmaking
process.

In the case of a patient without decisionmaking capacity, this
discussion should involve a surrogate for the patient. If possible,
however, the health care professional and patient should talk
together even when the patient is clearly incapable of exercising
decisionmaking authority over treatment, or has fluctuating or
uncertain capacity. Even the patient without decisionmaking
capacity may be able to understand some of what the professional
has to say and may be able to express preferences. Respect for
persons, including persons without decisionmaking capacity,
means that any patient who can participate to any extent in
the decisionmaking process should be encouraged to do so.

Family members or concerned friends will often be on the
scene and involved in discussions; patients typically welcome
their participation. Patients nonetheless are entitled to privacy
and confidentiality and have a right to forbid discussion with
family and friends. The responsible health care professional
should ascertain the patient's preference.
[*See also* **Ventilators,** *p. 39;* **Dialysis,** *p. 41;* **CPR,** *p. 48;* **Bleeding,**
p. 52; **Nutrition,** *p. 60;* **Antibiotics,** *p. 66*]

(3) Identifying the key decisionmaker. Many decisions about
life-sustaining treatment will emerge quite naturally from the
discussion process described above. Everyone involved may agree
about the best course of action. However, when the patient has
the capacity to decide about the treatment, it is the patient who
is the key decisionmaker, with the power to give binding consent
or refusal. When the patient lacks the capacity, the key
decisionmaker is someone else, a surrogate. Accordingly, the
responsible health care professional will identify the key
decisionmaker by determining whether the patient lacks

decisionmaking capacity. Section (a) below elaborates on assessing capacity.

When the patient lacks capacity, the health care professional will go on to identify a surrogate decisionmaker for the patient, as described below in Section (b). Sometimes there may not be a single surrogate; a number of family members and concerned others may be involved in the decisionmaking process. When that is the case, the responsible health care professional should discuss the treatment decision with these individuals in order to allow them to reach a conclusion on how to proceed. (See the standards for surrogate decisionmaking set forth in Section (4) (c), p. 27.) However, if the group cannot reach a consensus about the treatment decision, then it will be necessary to identify a single surrogate.

In specifying the key decisionmaker, we do not recommend isolating that person from others. The decisionmaker does not act alone. The responsible health care professional and often other members of the health care team, as well as family and concerned friends, are crucial to the decisionmaking process.

(a) Assessing decisionmaking capacity. A patient has the capacity to make the treatment decision when he or she can understand the relevant information, reflect on it in accordance with his or her values, and communicate with caregivers. A patient need not have decisionmaking capacity for all purposes in order to have the capacity to make the decision at hand. Some people have the capacity to make one choice but not another. Patients should be presumed to have the capacity to decide about treatment, unless it is determined that they lack it. (See PART SIX: Section III for further discussion of capacity.)

The responsible health care professional should ensure that the assessment of a patient's decisionmaking capacity is properly conducted. This is an important responsibility. It may require consultation with others. Health care institutions should develop policy on how to assess capacity within the institution, and might decide upon even more safeguards than these Guidelines recommend. The patient should be notified, whenever he or she might understand, that a surrogate will be exercising decisionmaking authority and that the patient or others can challenge the determination of lack of capacity. (See Section (8) (a), p. 31.)

Once the responsible health care professional determines that the patient lacks decisionmaking capacity, the professional should assess whether there are ways to restore capacity. In some cases, lack of capacity may have a reversible cause, such as over-medication, pain, dehydration, or metabolic abnormalities. The

professional should attempt to restore the patient's capacity prior to decisionmaking if possible.
[*See also* **Ventilators,** *p. 39*]

(b) Identifying a surrogate. When the patient lacks decision-making capacity, he or she should participate in the treatment decision as fully as possible; someone else, though, must serve as the ultimate source of consent or refusal. The responsible health care professional should identify this surrogate decisionmaker in consultation with other members of the health care team.

In identifying a surrogate, the professional should first honor any surrogate choice the patient has made—whether by advance directive or other written or oral statement. (See PART THREE.) The professional should also recognize the authority of a surrogate appointed by a court when the appointed surrogate's powers include medical decisionmaking. (If a court has appointed one such person, but the patient has designated someone else, the professional should seek legal advice to determine which is the appropriate surrogate—unless the two agree on a treatment decision so that deciding between them becomes unnecessary.) If the patient has made no choice and there is no court-appointed surrogate, then the goal is to find the person who is most involved with the patient and most knowledgeable about the patient's present and past feelings and preferences. Thus the responsible health care professional will usually identify one of the following as the surrogate:

1. the person designated by the patient through an advance directive or any other written or oral statement (see PART THREE);

2. a court-appointed surrogate, if the treatment decision in question is within the scope of the surrogate's authority (although this paragraph should not be construed to recommend such appointment); or

3. if neither of the above exists, the patient's spouse, a son or daughter, a parent, a brother or sister, or a concerned friend (in no priority order), as long as the surrogate is an adult, *i.e.*, has reached the age of majority in that state—usually 18 or 21. Immediate family members should be notified of the designation of a surrogate with lesser or no kinship.

(c) The patient who lacks a ready surrogate. One of the most difficult problems in medical decisionmaking is to whom to turn when the patient lacks decisionmaking capacity but has no one available and willing to act as surrogate. Various unsatisfactory ways of dealing with this have arisen, including waiting until the patient's medical condition worsens into an emergency so that consent to treat is implied by law and no surrogate is needed, or having the health care professional unilaterally decide for the patient. The first compromises patient care by waiting for a crisis and allows no orderly consideration of a decision to forgo treatment. The second compromises patient autonomy by leaving the decision in the hands of a person who may not know the patient's values. It also raises reasonable public concern, because there is no review and accountability for the decision that is made.

No decisionmaking mechanism is widely available to find attentive surrogates for the many people without them. There is also as yet no consensus on the proper solution. Some institutions and states are experimenting with a variety of mechanisms. Possibilities include some or all of the following: An institution, community agency, or other concerned provider organization could create a "surrogates committee" to provide a surrogate decisionmaker for each patient without capacity who lacks one. The responsible health care professional or health care institution could petition for a court-appointed guardian with authority to make health care decisions for each person without capacity and without a surrogate, a process that is costly, time-consuming, and public, but protective of civil rights and of the patient's estate. The state could permit ombudsmen functioning in state programs to provide ongoing personal advocacy for patients without capacity and with no surrogates, or to provide oversight for surrogates generated by surrogates committees. States, counties, or cities could establish Public Fiduciaries (or Public Guardians) who would investigate cases of possible incapacity and recommend appropriate court orders, including orders to provide ongoing representation for those with no surrogate. Courts could name private corporations as guardians; the corporations could provide services to the incapacitated patient while limiting the burden to the patient's representative, and could be required to adhere to regulatory or court-mandated standards.

Some combination of these kinds of procedures could create a surrogate for each patient, and provide the protection of institutional and public review of the surrogate's decisions. Some of these procedures may, however, be cumbersome and time-consuming. Whatever mechanisms are developed, each patient without decisionmaking capacity should have someone acting as his or her surrogate. Once a surrogate is put in place for a patient who lacked one, the surrogate should adhere to the same procedures and standards as other surrogates.

Some maintain that this kind of surrogate, who is not a family member or concerned friend of the patient, but may instead be a stranger, should have more limited discretion than a family or friend surrogate and perhaps should be subject to closer review. No wide agreement exists on this, however, or on the standards and mechanisms that would be used to further confine the discretion of a "stranger surrogate." We recommend that surrogates appointed for patients who lack them at least be held to the standards applied to family or friend surrogates, the standards set forth in Section (4) (c), p. 27. The fact that the surrogate may not know the patient well may play a part in others' evaluations of the surrogate.

To summarize our recommendations:

1. Appropriate mechanisms need to be developed to make decisions for patients without decisionmaking capacity who lack surrogates, and to review those decisions.

2. Each health care institution should adopt a written procedure for decisionmaking about life-sustaining treatment when a patient lacks capacity and has no surrogate.

3. Someone other than the patient's responsible health care professional should preferably act as surrogate, unless the patient has previously designated the professional to act as surrogate. Even when the professional is vigorously promoting the patient's well-being, it is important to have another person participating, whose primary function is to make choices as the patient would if he or she were able. If it is not possible for someone other than the responsible professional to act as surrogate, the professional should seek review of decisions to forgo life-sustaining treatment by the institutional ethics committee or other institutional mechanism for advising on ethical issues.

4. Some form of institutional review should be available for decisions about life-sustaining treatment for such patients, whether by a committee or by some other group or person within the institution.

(4) Making the decision.

(a) **The patient with decisionmaking capacity.** If the patient has decisionmaking capacity, then the patient is the ultimate judge of the benefits and burdens of a life-sustaining treatment, and whether the burdens outweigh the benefits. Individuals differ in what they see as a burden and a benefit, and in how they weigh the two against each other. To most people burdens include pain or suffering, hardships imposed on their loved ones, and financial cost. Most regard as benefits improved functioning, the relief of pain or suffering, the opportunity to live longer, and the chance to engage in satisfying activities.

Patients will usually find that life-sustaining treatment offers more benefits than burdens. In those cases, the treatment should be used. Some patients—particularly if they are terminally ill or suffering from an illness or disabling condition that is severe and irreversible—may decide that the burdens of a particular treatment outweigh the benefits, and choose to forgo that treatment. That choice should be honored. The responsible health care professional, however, should first discuss with the patient why he or she prefers to forgo treatment. Exploring the decision together is an important part of the process. If the patient is experiencing pain or suffering that can be ameliorated, the professional should discuss the possibility of amelioration to then see whether the patient still prefers to forgo treatment. The professional should make sure that the patient has not decided to forgo life-sustaining treatment in order to obtain relief from pain or suffering that can be alleviated without forgoing life-sustaining treatment.
[*See also* **Ventilators,** *p. 39;* **Dialysis,** *p. 41;* **Palliative Care,** *p. 73*]

(b) The patient whose capacity is fluctuating or uncertain. Some patients neither clearly possess nor clearly lack decisionmaking capacity; their capacity is fluctuating or uncertain. If the patient, responsible health care professional, and likely surrogate agree on the treatment decision, then there is no need to clarify the patient's capacity. When they do not agree or when no likely surrogate is on hand, and it is possible to adjust conditions or to delay the decision until the patient has decisionmaking capacity, that is the optimal course; the Guidelines above for patients with capacity then apply. If that is not possible, the Guidelines below for patients without decision-making capacity should apply instead.

(c) The patient who lacks decisionmaking capacity. When a patient lacks the capacity to make the treatment decision, so that a surrogate decisionmaker has decisionmaking authority instead, the surrogate should seek to choose as the patient would if he or she were able. Because the strength of the evidence of the patient's preferences will vary, the surrogate should apply one of the three different standards listed below. Whenever a surrogate can come to no clear view as to whether to forgo treatment, treatment should be administered; using the treatment on a trial basis with reevaluation after a set interval should be considered. (See Section (6) (a), p. 30.)

1. **Follow the patient's explicit directives.*** Where a patient who had decisionmaking capacity at the time, has left written directions in an advance directive (see PART THREE) or another form, or clear oral directions, and these directions seem intended to cover the situation presented, the surrogate should follow the directions.

2. **Or apply the patient's preferences and values.*** If the patient has left no directions about the treatment in question, the surrogate should apply what is known about the patient's preferences and values, trying to choose as the patient would have wanted.

3. **Or choose as a reasonable person in the patient's circumstances would.**** If there is not enough known about the patient's directions, preferences, and values to make an individualized decision, the surrogate should choose so as to promote the patient's interests as they would probably be conceived by a reasonable person in the patient's circumstances, selecting from within the range of choices that reasonable people would make. In order to flesh out this standard, we suggest below the major considerations involved in applying it to some important categories of patients:

   (i) **The patient who is terminally ill.** In applying the "reasonable person" standard to the terminally ill patient without decisionmaking capacity, the major considerations are usually whether forgoing treatment will allow the patient to avoid the burden of prolonged dying with pain or suffering, and whether the patient has the potential benefit of achieving some satisfaction if he or she survives longer.

   (ii) **The patient who has an illness or disabling condition that is severe and irreversible.** In applying the "reasonable person" standard to the patient with an illness or disabling condition that is severe and irreversible and who lacks decisionmaking capacity, the major consideration is the

---

*These are sometimes called a "substituted judgment" standard.
**This is sometimes called a "best interests" standard.

following: Would a reasonable person in the patient's circumstance probably prefer the termination of treatment because the patient's life is largely devoid of opportunities to achieve satisfaction, or full of pain or suffering with no corresponding benefits?

(iii) The patient with irreversible loss of consciousness. For the patient who has suffered an irreversible loss of consciousness, the major considerations in applying the "reasonable person" standard are somewhat different. Patients who are permanently unconscious are unaware of benefits or burdens. The only possible benefit to them of life-sustaining treatment is the possibility that the diagnosis of irreversible unconsciousness is wrong and they will regain consciousness. Accordingly, the major considerations are whether a reasonable person in the patient's circumstance would find that this benefit, as well as the benefits to the patient's family and concerned friends (such as satisfaction in caring for the patient and the meaningfulness of the patient's continued survival) are outweighed by the burdens on those loved ones (such as financial cost or emotional suffering).

(**The above list in no way suggests that treatment should be forgone just because a person falls into one of these categories;** nor does it mean that treatment may not be terminated for other patients.)
[*See also* **Bleeding,** *p. 52;* **Antibiotics,** *p. 66;* **Palliative Care,** *p. 73*]

(5) Documenting the decision. The use of most life-sustaining treatments requires a signed order; this is an accepted part of medical practice. When a decision has been made to withhold or withdraw a specific life-sustaining treatment, it is also advisable to put the appropriate signed orders and documentation in the patient's records. A decision to forgo such treatment is an important part of a patient's treatment plan, and without documentation the decision may not be known and followed. Documentation is also most likely to protect the interests of all involved, by promoting adherence to the decision, providing explanation, and allowing for orderly review when needed.

When a decision has been made to forgo an emergency life-sustaining treatment, such as cardiopulmonary resuscitation, it is imperative to write an order and document the decision. Otherwise, there is a serious risk that in an emergency the treatment will be administered to the patient.

The order and documentation should be signed by the patient's responsible health care professional (or another caregiver as authorized by institutional policy), though other members of the health care team may find it appropriate to add further notes and documentation. The general elements of the order and documentation should be clearly stated in institutional policy.
[*See also* **Ventilators,** *p. 39;* **CPR,** *p. 48;* **Bleeding,** *p. 52;* **Antibiotics,** *p. 66;* **Palliative Care,** *p. 73*]

(6) Implementing the decision.

(a) Time-limited trials. When possible, the responsible health care professional should present to the patient or surrogate the option of starting or continuing a particular life-sustaining treatment on a trial basis, with reevaluation after a specific time. Having a trial period may make it easier to evaluate a life-sustaining treatment if the effectiveness, benefits, or burdens are difficult to assess in advance. It is ethically preferable to try a treatment and to withdraw it if it fails, than not to try it at all. A trial period may reduce the patient's fears of losing control of a treatment and being "stuck on machines." It may also reduce emotional distress if a decision is later made to forgo the treatment. Time-limited trials will be impossible, however, in the case of some treatments, as noted where relevant in PART TWO.
[*See also* **CPR,** *p. 48;* **Nutrition,** *p. 60*]

(b) Supportive care. When a life-sustaining treatment is forgone, and whenever a patient is dying, the treatment team has an obligation to provide supportive care, to make the patient as comfortable as possible, and to assure the patient that adequate symptom control and support will be provided. Health care institutions and financers also have a responsibility for seeing that this occurs. Such care may include a wide variety of measures to provide symptomatic relief, sedation and pain control, skin care, and turning and positioning. If relieving the patient's pain or suffering requires sedation to the point of unconsciousness, it is ethically acceptable to do so with the patient's or surrogate's consent.
[*See also* **Ventilators,** *p. 39;* **Nutrition,** *p. 60;* **Antibiotics,** *p. 66;* **Palliative Care,** *p. 73*]

(c) Maximal therapeutic care. A decision to forgo one kind of life-sustaining treatment does not imply that the patient is forgoing any other forms of treatment. Forgoing one life-sustaining treatment is compatible with maximal therapeutic care of other types.
[*See also* **Ventilators,** *p. 39;* **CPR,** *p. 48*]

(d) **Stress and communication.** Health care professionals may sometimes find it stressful to care for dying or seriously ill patients, particularly when a life-sustaining treatment is forgone. There is a need for continual communication among the treatment team, patient, surrogate if any, and others who are involved. Any or all of these persons may need support; assistance from relevant professionals (including clergy) should be sought as required.

As we discuss in Section (8)(d), p. 32, nurses and physicians have independent ethical duties to patients, but decisions to forgo life-sustaining treatment may place special burdens on nurses. Nursing care (such as bathing, feeding, and toileting) is highly personal and involves intimate contact with the patient. Nurses may experience difficulty in implementing decisions to forgo treatment when they have formed a close attachment to the patient. Yet nurses usually play an important role in implementation, because forgoing life-sustaining treatment often demands particularly attentive nursing care. Nurses therefore need ways to discuss the consequences that such decisions have for their practice. Health care institutions should ensure that such ways exist.
[*See also* **CPR**, *p. 48;* **Bleeding**, *p. 52;* **Antibiotics**, *p. 66*]

(7) Changing the decision. A patient with decisionmaking capacity may change his or her decision concerning a life-sustaining treatment at any time. The surrogate for a patient without decisionmaking capacity may at any time change the decision concerning a life-sustaining treatment, provided that the change is in keeping with the Guidelines in Section (4)(c) above, p. 27. The change, and the reasons for it, should be documented in the patient's medical records.

(8) Objections and challenges.

(a) **Challenging the determination of lack of capacity.** The patient and involved others should be able to challenge a determination that the patient lacks decisionmaking capacity, pursuing the challenge through the institutional ethics committee or other institutional mechanism for advising on ethical issues, and through judicial review if necessary. Review should be prompt. If possible, no treatment decision should be effectuated until the challenge has been resolved. If, however, a treatment decision must be made in the interim, then if the challenge is made by the patient or surrogate, the patient should be assumed to have capacity and the patient should make the decision; otherwise, the responsible health care professional's determination of capacity should govern.

(b) **Challenging a surrogate.** If the patient without capacity or any involved person, including the responsible health care professional, challenges the identification of the surrogate or the surrogate's decision, then the challenge should be referred to the institutional ethics committee or other institutional mechanism for advising on ethical issues. Judicial review may also be necessary.

(c) **Futility.** In the event that the patient or surrogate requests a treatment that the responsible health care professional regards as clearly futile in achieving its physiological objective and so offering no physiological benefit to the patient, the professional has no obligation to provide it. However, the health care professional's value judgment that although a treatment will produce physiological benefit, the benefit is not sufficient to warrant the treatment, should not be used as a basis for determining a treatment to be futile. Treatment that is physiologically futile may offer psychological benefits and so may be warranted. The professional, patient, or surrogate may wish to consult with other health care professionals as well in assessing the futility of a treatment. The patient or surrogate should be at liberty to engage another health care professional.

(d) **Disagreement on the health care team.** Physicans and nurses intimately involved in the patient's care may sometimes question whether some aspect of the decisionmaking process has fallen short of what is ethically appropriate. Physicians and nurses have independent duties to assure that patients or surrogates have made fully informed decisions regarding the termination of treatment. Should disagreements about ethical concerns arise, they should be discussed with the responsible health care professional. If they cannot be resolved, they should be referred to the institutional ethics committee or other institutional mechanism for advising on ethical issues. Judicial review may also be necessary.

(e) **Withdrawal of health care professional or institution.** If a health care professional has serious objections to the decision of the patient or surrogate, so that carrying it out is impossible as a matter of conscience or commitment to principle, the professional is not obligated to do so. In such cases:

1. When the objecting professional is the responsible health care professional, he or she should inform the patient or surrogate of the problem and of the options that exist for transfer to another health care professional or institution. If the patient or surrogate decides to transfer, the professional should assist in an orderly process. If the patient

or surrogate prefers to transfer, but transfer is impossible (for example, because no other professional will accept the patient), the situation should be referred to the institutional ethics committee or other institutional mechanism for advising on ethical issues. Judicial review may also be necessary.

2. When the professional who objects to the decision is a member of the health care team but not the responsible health care professional, he or she should seek to be removed from the case in an orderly manner. The health care institution should attempt to accommodate the request.

Some health care institutions also have formal commitments to special principles, either religious or secular. These may prompt the institution to object to certain courses of action that a patient or surrogate has chosen. The right of such an institution to object or withdraw may be more limited by law than the right of individual health care professionals. Legal advice should be sought. Attempts to resolve the matter may involve resorting to the institutional ethics committee or another institutional mechanism for advising on ethical issues, and ultimately, if necessary, the courts. Institutions that do not provide certain treatments or that restrict patients' options to forgo treatment should notify patients and surrogates of this as early as possible, preferably before admission and in writing. An institution should not resist transfer of the patient, if the patient or surrogate wishes to exercise treatment options not allowed within it. [*See also* **Bleeding,** *p. 52*]

(9) Special comments.

(a) **Children.** When the patient is a child there are special considerations. These Guidelines do not present all of them, but rather a key amendment to the decisionmaking process recommended above, namely, that the child plays a different role than an adult in the process of consent or refusal. By "child" we mean minors, except those that state law treats as adults for the purpose of making these sorts of treatment decisions. Recall that these Guidelines only address patients beyond infancy.

Because they are minors, children cannot give legally recognized consent or refusal to treatment; generally their parents (or legal guardians) do instead. Consequently, the Guidelines above on patients without capacity obtain. (See Section (4)(c), p. 27.) Many children, however, are capable of participating in the decisionmaking process. Such a child should be allowed to participate as much as possible. A child who can express assent or objection to a treatment choice should be encouraged to do so. If the parents or other surrogate make a treatment choice contrary to the child's preference, the responsible health care professional should explore with the child and parents or other surrogate the basis for the disagreement, and should attempt to resolve it. Resort to an institutional ethics committee or other institutional mechanism for advising on ethical issues may be necessary. Judicial review may also be necessary.

[*See also* **Ventilators,** *p. 39;* **Dialysis,** *p. 41;* **CPR,** *p. 48;* **Bleeding,** *p. 52;* **Nutrition,** *p. 60;* **Palliative Care,** *p. 73*]

PART TWO:
Specific Treatment Modalities

Section A.
GUIDELINES ON LONG-TERM
LIFE-SUPPORTING TECHNOLOGY —
VENTILATORS AND DIALYSIS

I. INTRODUCTION

II. GUIDELINES ON VENTILATORS

[NOTE: These Guidelines on ventilators build on PART ONE. Sections not underlined below are found in PART ONE and apply here without amendment. Where a section is underlined, amendments or additions to that section of PART ONE appear here.]

(1) Underlying ethical values
    (a) Patient well-being—benefiting more than burdening the patient
    (b) Patient self-determination
    (c) The ethical integrity of health care professionals
    (d) Justice or equity

(2) Evaluation and discussion
    (a) Evaluating the patient
    (b) Facilitating discussion

(3) Identifying the key decisionmaker
    (a) Assessing decisionmaking capacity
    (b) Identifying a surrogate
    (c) The patient who lacks a ready surrogate

(4) Making the decision
    (a) The patient with decisionmaking capacity
    (b) The patient whose capacity is fluctuating or uncertain
    (c) The patient who lacks decisionmaking capacity

(5) Documenting the decision

(6) Implementing the decision
    (a) Time-limited trials
    (b) Supportive care
    (c) Maximal therapeutic care
    (d) Stress and communication

(7) Changing the decision

(8) Objections and challenges
    (a) Challenging the determination of lack of capacity
    (b) Challenging a surrogate
    (c) Futility
    (d) Disagreement on the health care team
    (e) Withdrawal of health care professional or institution

(9) Special comments
    (a) Children
    (b) Weaning

III. GUIDELINES ON DIALYSIS

[NOTE: These Guidelines on dialysis build on PART ONE. Sections not underlined below are found in PART ONE and apply here without amendment. Where a section is underlined, amendments or additions to that section of PART ONE appear here.]

(1) Underlying ethical values
    (a) Patient well-being—benefiting more than burdening the patient
    (b) Patient self-determination
    (c) The ethical integrity of health care professionals
    (d) Justice or equity

(2) Evaluation and discussion
    (a) Evaluating the patient
    (b) Facilitating discussion

(3) Identifying the key decisionmaker
    (a) Assessing decisionmaking capacity
    (b) Identifying a surrogate
    (c) The patient who lacks a ready surrogate

(4) Making the decision
    (a) The patient with decisionmaking capacity
    (b) The patient whose capacity is fluctuating or uncertain
    (c) The patient who lacks decisionmaking capacity

(5) Documenting the decision

(6) Implementing the decision
    (a) Time-limited trials
    (b) Supportive care
    (c) Maximal therapeutic care
    (d) Stress and communication

(7) Changing the decision

(8) Objections and challenges
    (a) Challenging the determination of lack of capacity
    (b) Challenging a surrogate
    (c) Futility
    (d) Disagreement on the health care team
    (e) Withdrawal of health care professional or institution

(9) Special comments
    (a) Children
    (b) <u>Integrated decisionmaking process</u>
    (c) <u>Place of death</u>
    (d) <u>Incentives</u>

PART TWO:
Specific Treatment Modalities

Section A.
GUIDELINES ON THE USE OF LONG-TERM
LIFE-SUPPORTING TECHNOLOGY—
VENTILATORS AND DIALYSIS

I. INTRODUCTION

Using a life-sustaining technology over an extended period of time can raise substantial ethical issues. Two such long-term life-supporting technologies currently causing widely perceived ethical challenges are ventilators and dialysis. Patients and others may fear that once the patient "gets on" such a technology, the patient will not be able to "get off." There may indeed be substantial barriers, particularly psychological ones, to stopping ventilator use or dialysis, even at the patient's behest.

Yet a patient should be able to refuse even treatment he or she has been receiving for an extended period of time. In the INTRODUCTION and PART SIX of these Guidelines, we discuss withholding and withdrawing treatment. There we argue that treatment can ethically be withdrawn whenever it can ethically be withheld. Decisions to stop treatment—like decisions not to begin treatment in the first place—should rest on whether the burdens of treatment and the life it offers exceed the benefits from the patient's perspective. Patients should consequently be entitled to stop either ventilator use or dialysis.

The Guidelines below on ventilators concern decisions on whether to stop the treatment, plus decisions on whether to start ventilation when there is enough time to go through a deliberate decisionmaking process. This Section, however, does not concern the emergency initiation of ventilation, which is the most frequent way that this treatment begins. That is covered in PART TWO: Section B on cardiopulmonary resuscitation.

Patients and their surrogates, if any, should participate in decisions about whether to start or stop ventilator use. Anecdotal information suggests that in the past, some patients have been removed from the ventilator without consultation of the patient or surrogate, or the ventilator has been adjusted so that it delivered inadequate ventilation and oxygenation to the patient without such consultation. We strongly reject both practices.

In contrast to ventilator use, the need to start dialysis is usually anticipated, and there is an opportunity to decide in advance whether to use the treatment at all. There is also, of course, an opportunity to decide to stop dialysis once begun and stopping is probably not uncommon. Since dialysis is an intermittent treatment, a decision can be made at numerous points to stop by simply not undertaking further treatment.

Two aspects of dialysis are distinctive for the purposes of these Guidelines. First, dialysis may take place not only in the hospital, nursing home, or other large health care institution, but also in the outpatient center or the home. Consequently, the possibility of terminating dialysis may first arise outside of a medical institution that is prepared to ensure a full evaluation and provide immediate response and support. Second, the dialysis patient who is a renal transplant candidate sometimes considers stopping dialysis without the transplant; this raises issues that are different than those facing the patient who is not transplantable. We consider both of these aspects in the Guidelines that follow.

II. GUIDELINES ON VENTILATORS

[REMEMBER: The Guidelines below are amendments and additions to the corresponding sections of PART ONE. They must be read together with PART ONE.]

(1) **Underlying ethical values.**

(c) **The ethical integrity of health care professionals.** A health care professional should not pretend to use the ventilator properly while intentionally using it inadequately. The professional should also not remove the patient from the ventilator in a way that is expected to prompt the patient's death while purporting to wean the patient. The professional should remove a patient from a ventilator only with the patient's or surrogate's permission, and should not request other health care personnel to carry out a decision that he or she would not personally carry out.

(2) **Evaluation and discussion.**

(b) **Facilitating discussion.** The health care professional may encounter special obstacles to discussion when the patient is on a ventilator, because the patient may not be able to speak. Health care professionals should attempt to establish other ways for the patient to communicate, such as writing, using an alphabet board, nodding or head shaking, or using electronic devices to vocalize. If the patient cannot engage in discussion, the health care professional should nonetheless talk to the patient, who may be able to signal some kind of response or simply listen.

(3) Identifying the key decisionmaker.

(a) **Assessing decisionmaking capacity.** Assessing a patient's decisionmaking capacity may be difficult if the patient cannot speak because of the ventilator. Health care professionals should try to establish communication using methods such as those suggested above. However, an overwhelming inability to communicate may itself render the patient effectively incapable of making the treatment decision, because part of decisionmaking capacity is the ability to communicate the choice.

(4) Making the decision.

(a) **The patient with decisionmaking capacity.** Particularly in the case of ventilator use, the patient who expresses the desire to stop the treatment may be responding to physical and psychological discomfort that may be alleviated by adjusting the ventilator or by some other means. The health care professional should investigate this possibility with the patient, obtaining appropriate consultations. They may agree on trying to ameliorate the discomfort to see whether the patient then would choose to continue ventilator use.

(5) Documenting the decision.
In part because of concerns that in the past ventilator use has sometimes been discontinued without the patient's or surrogate's consent, it is important that every decision to withdraw ventilation be documented and that an order be written.

(6) Implementing the decision.

(b) **Supportive care.** Ventilator use routinely requires nursing care and respiratory therapy, including suctioning, hyperventilation, and turning the patient. It is ethically acceptable to sedate the patient if necessary to insure comfort. If relieving the patient's dyspnea or other discomfort requires sedation to the point of unconsciousness, it is ethically acceptable to do so with the patient's or surrogate's consent.

(c) **Maximal therapeutic care.** Ventilator use often occurs in the Intensive Care Unit, where a number of life-sustaining treatments may frequently be used. A decision by the patient or surrogate to use the ventilator should not be construed as acceptance of all forms of life-sustaining treatment. The responsible health care professional should discuss other relevant forms of life-sustaining treatment with the patient or surrogate to allow them to make decisions about those other treatments.

(9) Special comments.

(b) **Weaning.** Generally, whenever the health care professional believes that weaning the patient from the ventilator may prove successful, the professional should attempt it. In some cases, however, the patient or surrogate may decide to forgo ventilator use and may wish to decline attempts at weaning because the decision about ventilation is part of a fundamental decision to forgo any life-sustaining treatment.

III. GUIDELINES ON DIALYSIS

[REMEMBER: The Guidelines below are amendments and additions to the corresponding sections of PART ONE. They must be read together with PART ONE.].

(2) Evaluation and discussion.

(a) **Evaluating the patient.** When a patient or surrogate is considering whether to forgo dialysis, it is essential that the patient be fully and promptly evaluated by the responsible health care professional, even if the patient is not an in-patient in a medical institution. Because dialysis is frequently supervised most directly by personnel other than the responsible health care professional, it is important that all such personnel participate in the evaluation process.

(b) **Facilitating discussion.** A vital part of discussing whether to forgo dialysis is addressing the patient's transplantation options. In order to make an informed decision about whether to forgo dialysis, the patient or surrogate must receive an evaluation of whether the patient is transplantable and, if so, what the transplantation possibilities are and what transplantation involves.

(4) Making the decision.

(a) **The patient with decisonmaking capacity.** It is important to explore with patients already on dialysis why they wish to stop the treatment. A number of aspects of dialysis have the potential for discouraging a patient from continuing. It may be that the patient's discomforts can be ameliorated without stopping the treatment entirely. This should be discussed with the patient.

(9) Special comments.

(b) **Integrated decisionmaking process.** Initiating some forms of dialysis requires a surgical procedure, which cannot be performed without informed consent. In such cases, the patient's or surrogate's decision on whether to give consent for the surgery and the decision to undertake or forgo dialysis should occur as part of a single decisionmaking process.

(c) **Place of death.** Because dialysis may be performed in an outpatient center or at home, the health care professional and the patient or surrogate should address the question of where death will occur when a decision has been made to forgo dialysis. Often a patient will wish to die in the hospital, where supportive and palliative care are readily available. If the patient wishes to die at home, the health care professional should inform the patient and caregivers of the risks and burdens, and of the options for supportive care at home. The patient's preference concerning the place of death should ordinarily control, as long as adequate care can be arranged.

(d) **Incentives.** The nature of reimbursement incentives should not be allowed to influence decisions on whether to stop dialysis.

PART TWO:
Specific Treatment Modalities
Section B.
GUIDELINES ON EMERGENCY
INTERVENTIONS—CARDIOPULMONARY
RESUSCITATION (CPR) AND TREATMENT FOR
LIFE-THREATENING BLEEDING

I. INTRODUCTION

II. GUIDELINES ON CARDIOPULMONARY
RESUSCITATION (CPR)

[NOTE: These Guidelines on cardiopulmonary resuscitation build on PART ONE. Sections not underlined below are found in PART ONE and apply here without amendment. Where a section is underlined, amendments or additions to that section of PART ONE appear here.]

(1) Underlying ethical values
   (a) Patient well-being—benefiting more than burdening the patient
   (b) Patient self-determination
   (c) The ethical integrity of health care professionals
   (d) Justice or equity

(2) Evaluation and discussion
   (a) Evaluating the patient
   (b) Facilitating discussion

(3) Identifying the key decisionmaker
   (a) Assessing decisionmaking capacity
   (b) Identifying a surrogate
   (c) The patient who lacks a ready surrogate

(4) Making the decision
   (a) The patient with decisionmaking capacity
   (b) The patient whose capacity is fluctuating or uncertain
   (c) The patient who lacks decisionmaking capacity

(5) Documenting the decision

(6) Implementing the decision
   (a) Time-limited trials
   (b) Supportive care
   (c) Maximal therapeutic care

(d) <u>Stress and communication</u>

(7) Changing the decision

(8) Objections and challenges
    (a) Challenging the determination of lack of capacity
    (b) Challenging a surrogate
    (c) Futility
    (d) Disagreement on the health care team
    (e) Withdrawal of health care professional or institution

(9) Special comments
    (a) Children
    (b) <u>Periodic review of DNR order</u>
    (c) <u>Presumption in favor of providing CPR</u>
    (d) <u>Interinstitutional transfers</u>
    (e) <u>Emergency medical service CPR</u>
    (f) <u>Adoption of DNR policy</u>
    (g) <u>Reimbursement, admission, and transfer</u>

III. GUIDELINES ON TREATMENT FOR LIFE-THREATENING BLEEDING

[NOTE: These Guidelines on treatment for life-threatening bleeding build on PART ONE. Sections not underlined below are found in PART ONE and apply here without amendment. Where a section is underlined, amendments or additions to that section of PART ONE appear here.]

(1) Underlying ethical values
    (a) Patient well-being—benefiting more than burdening the patient
    (b) <u>Patient self-determination</u>
    (c) The ethical integrity of health care professionals
    (d) <u>Justice or equity</u>

(2) Evaluation and discussion
    (a) <u>Evaluating the patient</u>
    (b) <u>Facilitating discussion</u>

(3) Identifying the key decisionmaker
    (a) Assessing decisionmaking capacity
    (b) Identifying a surrogate
    (c) The patient who lacks a ready surrogate

(4) Making the decision
    (a) The patient with decisionmaking capacity
    (b) The patient whose capacity is fluctuating or uncertain

(c) <u>The patient who lacks decisionmaking capacity</u>

(5) <u>Documenting the decision</u>

(6) Implementing the decision
  (a) Time-limited trials
  (b) Supportive care
  (c) Maximal therapeutic care
  (d) <u>Stress and communication</u>

(7) Changing the decision

(8) Objections and challenges
  (a) Challenging the determination of lack of capacity
  (b) Challenging a surrogate
  (c) Futility
  (d) Disagreement on the health care team
  (e) <u>Withdrawal of health care professional or institution</u>

(9) Special comments
  (a) <u>Children</u>
  (b) <u>The patient who is pregnant or has dependent children</u>
  (c) <u>Presumption in favor of providing treatment for bleeding</u>
  (d) <u>Adoption of policy</u>

PART TWO:
Specific Treatment Modalities

Section B.
GUIDELINES ON EMERGENCY
INTERVENTIONS—CARDIOPULMONARY
RESUSCITATION (CPR) AND TREATMENT FOR
LIFE-THREATENING BLEEDING

I. INTRODUCTION

Emergency treatment raises special ethical issues. In a life-threatening emergency there is no time to go through an extended decisionmaking process. Ethically there is a traditional presumption in favor of preserving life when no decision has been made to forgo the treatment in question, and legally there is a presumption of patient consent to treatment in an emergency. In some cases, however, an emergency can be anticipated; then the patient or surrogate should have an opportunity to consider ahead of time whether the treatment is desired. In addition, whenever there is some reason to question whether the patient or surrogate wishes the emergency treatment, health care professionals should inquire before the emergency to determine whether the presumption of consent is valid. A refusal of future emergency treatment is a revocation of the otherwise presumed consent.

If emergency treatment is to be forgone, that should be clearly established in advance so no time is wasted in confusion at the moment of crisis. When doubt exists over whether a decision to forgo treatment has been properly made, treatment to preserve life should be given. Because a decision to refuse an emergency intervention should thus occur before the crisis, this Section amends the basic Decisionmaking Process of PART ONE more than any other Section of PART TWO.

These Guidelines cover two emergency treatments: cardiopulmonary resuscitation (CPR) and treatment for bleeding. By "CPR" we do not refer to the efforts of the person on the street to revive someone who has collapsed. Instead, we refer to treatment administered by health care professionals for cardiac or respiratory arrest. This is the subject of most guidelines to date on forgoing life-sustaining treatment. Many hospitals now have such guidelines in place, and "do not resuscitate" (DNR) guidelines for nursing homes and emergency medical services have been reported as well.

The propriety of DNR orders—with certain procedural safeguards and limitations—is now widely acknowledged. Although

CPR restores functioning in a significant number of cases, in many cases it either fails entirely, or forestalls death but leaves the patient unconscious or quite disabled. Moreover, CPR is invasive and may seem violent, facts that may give the patient or surrogate pause. Consequently, it has been recognized increasingly that patients—especially those who are terminally ill—may wish to forgo CPR.

The Guidelines that follow recommend that the responsible health care professional discuss CPR and the option of a DNR order with certain categories of patients or their surrogates. We focus on these categories because these are either patients for whom an arrest is anticipated—giving an opportunity to check the presumption of consent to emergency treatment—or patients for whom the presumption of consent to CPR may reasonably be questioned. Any other patients who wish to make a decision about CPR should be allowed to do so. In the absence of a DNR order, resuscitation should be attempted, unless it will clearly be futile in restoring cardiac and respiratory function.

These Guidelines distinguish decisions concerning resuscitation from decisions concerning other aspects of care. A patient with metastatic cancer, for instance, might well decide to fight the disease with all interventions available. But the patient may at the same time decide that, if there is deterioration to the point of cardiac or respiratory arrest, he or she does not want CPR administered. As most DNR guidelines clearly state, having a DNR order is compatible with maximal therapeutic care.

The Guidelines on CPR also address the problem of emergency medical services, which routinely attempt resuscitation without knowing whether the patient has already refused CPR. This is a difficult problem, and we offer some suggestions.

This Section of the Guidelines covers treatment for life-threatening bleeding as well. Some patients may decide that in the event of life-threatening bleeding they want no corrective treatment; or they may wish to discontinue such treatment once begun. This most often arises with patients who are Jehovah's Witnesses.*

The Guidelines on bleeding differ from the Guidelines on CPR in a major respect. The Guidelines on CPR recommend that the health care professional talk to several categories of patients about forgoing treatment before a cardiac or respiratory arrest. However,

---

*Some members of other religious groups may also refuse blood and blood products for religious reasons. Our references to Jehovah's Witnesses should be taken to include those other groups.

the Guidelines on bleeding recommend that professionals discuss the possibility of forgoing treatment in advance only when the patient is known to be a Jehovah's Witness or there is some other reason to question the presumption of the patient's consent to emergency transfusion for life-threatening bleeding. For other patients the Guidelines do not advocate discussion before the crisis (though the Guidelines would certainly permit it), but rather when the crisis occurs if there is enough time to go through an extended decisionmaking process or after the crisis to decide whether to stop treatment already begun. Since a bleeding problem often extends over time, a treatment decision can sometimes be made after emergency treatment and after the patient's condition has stabilized. Cardiac or respiratory arrest, on the other hand, is an acute, time-limited event, so that a decision to forgo CPR can only be made in advance of the crisis. In addition, people may question the desirability of CPR more often than the desirability of transfusion.

II. GUIDELINES ON CARDIOPULMONARY RESUSCITATION (CPR)

[REMEMBER: The Guidelines below are amendments and additions to the corresponding sections of PART ONE. They must be read together with PART ONE.]

(1) **Underlying ethical values.**

(c) **The ethical integrity of health care professionals.** "Show codes" and "slow codes"—appearing to provide CPR while not doing so, or doing so in a way that is known to be ineffective—compromise the ethical integrity of health care professionals and should be avoided. Such practices are incompatible with the ethical use of DNR orders. Unless there is documentation of a decision by the patient or surrogate and responsible health care professional to the contrary, any code called should be a full code. Specific limitations on CPR (such as "no intubation" or "no defibrillation") make successful resuscitation much less likely. Such limitations should consequently be exceedingly rare and should be used only if explicitly requested by a fully informed patient or surrogate.

(2) **Evaluation and discussion.**

(b) **Facilitating discussion.** The responsible health care professional should initiate a discussion concerning CPR and the option of a DNR order with the patient or the surrogate, whenever one of the following categories applies:

1. There is some reason to question the presumption of consent to CPR.

2. The patient is terminally ill.

3. The patient has an illness or disabling condition that is severe and irreversible.

4. The patient has suffered an irreversible loss of consciousness.

5. The patient is reasonably likely to have a cardiac or respiratory arrest.

(This does not mean that patients in the above categories should necessarily have a DNR order, but rather that the presumption of consent to CPR should be questioned in such cases, so that the patient or surrogate should have an opportunity to consent to or refuse CPR.) In addition to patients in these categories, the health care professional should hold such a discussion with any patient or surrogate who wishes to do so. Speaking to patients well in advance of a crisis, and having a policy requiring discussion with a range of patients, will help minimize the stress patients may experience from the discussion.

A patient's or surrogate's consent to an initial resuscitation should not be presumed to constitute consent to further resuscitations. After the initial resuscitation, the responsible health care professional should again consult with the patient or surrogate. (See also Section (6) (a), p. 50.)

Health care professionals should discuss DNR orders not only with patients in the hospital or nursing home, but also with patients before they require institutional care and with patients who will remain at home through their illness and dying. The best place for a DNR discussion is not the Emergency Room or Intensive Care Unit when the patient is already extremely debilitated, but in the ambulatory setting while the patient is still capable of making decisions about care. In some cases the discussion may have to be forgone in an emergency setting, especially when there is no reason to question the presumption of consent to CPR. In those cases, however, health care professionals should discuss the option of a DNR order with the patient or surrogate as soon as possible.

Whenever possible, the health care professional should use the occasion of the DNR discussion to discuss other aspects of the patient's care. At the same time that the patient or surrogate makes a decision about CPR, he or she should also be encouraged to make decisions about other treatments (ventilator use, dialysis, the use of blood and blood products, antibiotics, etc., as appropriate). However, the health care professional should make it clear that a patient or surrogate may refuse CPR but decide in favor of any or all other treatments.

(5) Documenting the decision. When a patient or surrogate has decided to forgo CPR, the responsible health care professional should write a DNR order. The health care institution should adopt a policy that specifies how DNR orders should be recorded. If either the patient or surrogate questions the desirability of a DNR order previously written, then until the matter is resolved, the patient's medical records should clearly show that no DNR order is currently in effect.

(6) Implementing the decision.

(a) Time-limited trials. These are not possible in the case of CPR, because of the nature of the crisis and treatment. It is possible, however, to use frequency trials, employing CPR but then evaluating its desirability for future use.

(c) Maximal therapeutic care. A DNR order should not be understood as an indication that other life-sustaining treatment should also be withheld or that the patient should not be admitted to the Intensive Care Unit. A DNR order is compatible with maximal therapeutic care and ICU admission.

(d) Stress and communication. Providing other life-sustaining or curative treatments to a patient with a DNR order may cause confusion and stress for any members of the treatment team who misunderstand a DNR order as an indication that other treatment should also be forgone. The responsible health care professional should discuss the DNR order and treatment plan with the entire team.

(9) Special comments.

(b) Periodic review of DNR order. For all patients in a health care institution, DNR orders should be reviewed at regular intervals by the responsible health care professional. He or she should reevaluate the patient, consult again with the patient or surrogate if there is any change, and rewrite the order if appropriate. The length of the interval between evaluations should be established by institutional policy. The policy should be rigorously enforced. DNR orders, however, should not automatically expire after a set period of time. Otherwise, patients may receive CPR purely because review of the order has been delayed for some reason and the order has consequently expired.

Similarly, when a patient with a DNR order is being treated on an ambulatory basis, the responsible health care professional should review the order at set intervals and alert the patient or surrogate to this. However, as discussed immediately below in Sections (d) and (e), a DNR order may not be effective outside of a residential health care institution.

(c) Presumption in favor of providing CPR. Any patient without a DNR order should receive CPR in the event of a cardiac or respiratory arrest. At the time of such an arrest, the health care professional may call off the resuscitation if the effort clearly cannot restore cardiac and respiratory function. (This might apply when treatment has been delayed for a prolonged period following arrest, when the patient is receiving full but ineffective treatment for failure of other organ systems in an ICU and then develops cardiac or respiratory arrest, or when the patient has severe acidosis.) Health care professionals and institutions must be vigilant not to allow this exception to justify failure to discuss the issues with the patient or surrogate in advance.

(d) Interinstitutional transfers. When a patient is transferred from one health care institution to another, both institutions should make sure that the DNR status established in the old institution is communicated to the new one. Soon after the patient's admission to the new institution, the responsible health care professional should discuss with the patient or surrogate the patient's resuscitative status. The professional should explain any relevant differences in the new institution and again establish the patient's resuscitative status. This should be documented in the patient's medical records. Institutions should explore with one another whether there is some way for a DNR order written in one setting to remain effective as the patient is transferred, though the review and reestablishment of resuscitative status in the new setting should occur in any event.

(e) Emergency medical service CPR. Emergency medical services (EMSs) face special problems with DNR orders. When called to a health care institution during an emergency, they cannot easily evaluate the propriety and authenticity of a DNR order. If they are called to the home, they cannot readily evaluate the patient's or family's spoken requests to refrain from using CPR. Means have to be established to communicate legitimate DNR orders and decisions to EMSs. We recommend that within each community, the EMSs, health care institutions, and local health care professionals collaborate to establish a workable DNR policy for EMSs, so that they may honor proper DNR orders, even in the home setting.

Until that has been accomplished, we recommend that an emergency medical service administer CPR to every patient undergoing an arrest, with one exception: When the service picks up the patient at a health care institution known to have a written DNR policy and is shown a DNR order signed by a health care professional, that order should be honored. This exception may raise problems for some EMSs, particularly those whose personnel take their orders from their own professional in a back-up center. However, the possibility of using this exception should be explored.

(f) Adoption of DNR policy. Health care institutions and emergency medical services should adopt written DNR policies in order to anticipate emergencies effectively and to ensure that health care personnel will know how to respond. The institution or service should educate health care personnel about the policy, monitor its effectiveness, and revise it as necessary. Formulating DNR policy has been one of the main activities of institutional ethics committees. (See PART FIVE: Section A (8), p. 103.)

(g) Reimbursement, admission, and transfer. A DNR order should not be used to categorize patients for purposes of reimbursement by health care financers. This might create financial pressures that would interfere with honoring the patient's wishes or surrogate's choice. A DNR order should also not be required or prohibited as a condition of admission or transfer to any health care institution or unit or service within an institution except hospices. Patients should not be forced to forgo one form of life-sustaining treatment to get other treatments and services.

II. GUIDELINES ON TREATMENT FOR LIFE-THREATENING BLEEDING

[REMEMBER: The Guidelines below are amendments and additions to the corresponding sections of PART ONE. They must be read together with PART ONE.]

(1) Underlying ethical values.

(b) Patient self-determination. Among the treatments a patient may choose to forgo is the administration of blood and blood products. This refusal arises most frequently on religious grounds, usually asserted by a Jehovah's Witness. Because an individual's freedom to act in accord with personal religious values is one aspect of autonomy, the right of a Jehovah's Witness to refuse blood should be recognized. However, as with non-religious aspects of autonomy, the right of self-determination is not absolute. In some cases, the Jehovah's Witness may not be ethically entitled to forgo life-sustaining treatment for bleeding. (See Sections (9)(a) and (b), p. 55.)

Some patients may refuse transfusions on non-religious grounds. The patient or surrogate may question whether the burdens to the patient, including the risks associated with transfusion, exceed the benefits, particularly when a patient requires transfusion repeatedly or has a terminal illness.

(d) Justice or equity. Blood and blood products are scarce resources, and blood banks as well as health care institutions may experience periodic shortages. Individual health care professionals should not create triage policies at the bedside restricting the access of individual patients to these resources. This would produce an undesirable conflict of interest, threatening the professional's loyalty to the patient. It also would make for inconsistent policies, not fully informed by the facts, and unavailable for public scrutiny. Instead, blood triage policy should be formulated by groups within the health care institution or blood bank, outside of the context of an individual patient's care, and should be written to allow review. (See also PART FIVE: Section C on Economic Considerations.)

(2) Evaluation and discussion.

(a) Evaluating the patient. The health care professional evaluating a patient who may wish to forgo blood and blood products should determine whether there are alternatives to the use of blood or blood products.

(b) Facilitating discussion. As soon as it becomes known that a patient is a Jehovah's Witness, whether in a health care institution or ambulatory setting, the responsible health care professional should initiate a discussion with the patient or surrogate concerning the use of blood and blood products. For these patients, a decision on whether blood and blood products will be used should be made in advance of life-threatening bleeding when possible. Similarly, when there is some other reason to question the presumption of a patient's or surrogate's consent to emergency treatment for life-threatening bleeding, the professional should initiate a discussion and a decision should be made before the crisis if possible. For all other patients the decisionmaking process may occur at any of several points: when serious bleeding is expected but has not yet started; when such bleeding occurs, if there is time to go through the entire decisionmaking process; or when treatment for bleeding has started and the question is whether to continue.

When the patient is a Jehovah's Witness, it may be necessary for the health care professional to speak to the patient alone in order to determine if the patient is refusing transfusion voluntarily. When the patient appears to be under pressure from family or others, he or she should be offered an opportunity to discuss the refusal of transfusion with a health care professional who is not directly involved in the case, in order to ensure a voluntary decision. In addition, sometimes a Jehovah's Witness may actually wish to have a court order override his or her religious refusal. The health care professional should attempt to find out whether this is the case.

(4) Making the decision.

(c) The patient who lacks decisionmaking capacity. When the patient without decisionmaking capacity is a Jehovah's Witness, there is only one acceptable basis for a religious refusal of transfusion by the surrogate: the patient, while he or she still had decisionmaking capacity, clearly and reliably expressed that he or she was a Jehovah's Witness and would not accept blood or blood products under these circumstances, and the patient has not subsequently contradicted this, either with or without decisionmaking capacity.

(5) Documenting the decision. Most hospitals and other health care facilities will probably request the Jehovah's Witness patient or the patient's surrogate to sign a document refusing blood and blood products. This should be supplemented by an order written by a health care professional.

(6) Implementing the decision.

(d) Stress and communication. A decision to forgo blood and blood products may cause confusion and stress for members of the treatment team, particularly when the patient is generally healthy and the decision is made on religious grounds. The responsible health care professional should discuss the matter with the entire team.

(8) Objections and challenges.

(e) Withdrawal of health care professional or institution. Some health care professionals may prefer not to take responsibility for a Jehovah's Witness patient who refuses blood and blood products. Health care institutions, particularly hospitals, should establish a list of health care professionals, especially surgeons and anesthesiologists, who are willing to treat such patients. This will facilitate the patient's transfer to an appropriate health care professional if the initial professional decides to withdraw.

(9) Special comments.

(a) Children. If the patient is a minor, the responsible health care professional should seek ethical and legal advice on whether the patient, parents, or a non-parental surrogate may decide to forgo treatment on religious grounds. A number of courts have concluded that parents cannot refuse blood and blood products for a child on religious grounds, because this may deprive the child of the opportunity to decide as an adult whether to adhere to that religious position. This same argument also supports a strong ethical presumption against parents' refusing blood or blood products for their children on religious grounds, though it is possible that in some special circumstances such a refusal might be ethically justified.

(b) The patient who is pregnant or has dependent children. When a patient who is a Jehovah's Witness is pregnant or has a dependent child, a refusal of blood and blood products may require consideration by the institutional ethics committee or other institutional mechanism for advising on ethical issues, and ultimately a judicial determination. This is because the right to forgo treatment may sometimes be restricted on the grounds that it will cause harm to specific others.

(c) Presumption in favor of providing treatment for bleeding. All patients should receive treatment for bleeding in an emergency, unless there is documentation in the medical record of a currently effective refusal of blood and blood products, or the patient, while capable of making decisions, has given written directions refusing blood and blood products under such circumstances, and the patient has not subsequently contradicted this. Once the patient has been treated and stabilized, the full decisionmaking process recommended in these Guidelines can be undertaken, if the patient or surrogate so desires.

(d) Adoption of policy. It is particularly important for hospitals to adopt written policy on the transfusion of Jehovah's Witnesses in order to anticipate emergencies effectively and ensure that health care personnel know what to do. The hospital should educate health care personnel about the policy, monitor its effectiveness, and revise it as necessary.

It is unclear whether Jehovah's Witnesses pose a substantial problem for health care institutions other than hospitals, such as nursing homes and hospices, as well as emergency medical services. In communities where such a problem exists, those institutions and EMSs should also develop policy, and should work out ways of communicating refusals of blood and blood products, when a patient is transferred from one institution to another. In developing policy, it may be useful to discuss the issues with local Jehovah's Witnesses, both clergy and laypersons.

PART TWO:
Specific Treatment Modalities
Section C.
GUIDELINES ON MEDICAL PROCEDURES FOR
SUPPLYING NUTRITION AND HYDRATION

I. INTRODUCTION

II. GUIDELINES ON MEDICAL PROCEDURES FOR SUPPLYING NUTRITION AND HYDRATION

[NOTE: These Guidelines on nutrition and hydration build on PART ONE. Sections not underlined below are found in PART ONE and apply here without amendment. Where a section is underlined, amendments or additions to that section of PART ONE appear here.]

(1) Underlying ethical values
  (a) Patient well-being—benefiting more than burdening the patient
  (b) Patient self-determination
  (c) The ethical integrity of health care professionals
  (d) Justice or equity

(2) Evaluation and discussion
  (a) <u>Evaluating the patient</u>
  (b) <u>Facilitating discussion</u>

(3) Identifying the key decisionmaker
  (a) Assessing decisionmaking capacity
  (b) Identifying a surrogate
  (c) The patient who lacks a ready surrogate

(4) Making the decision
  (a) The patient with decisionmaking capacity
  (b) The patient whose capacity is fluctuating or uncertain
  (c) The patient who lacks decisionmaking capacity

(5) Documenting the decision

(6) Implementing the decision
  (a) <u>Time-limited trials</u>
  (b) <u>Supportive care</u>
  (c) Maximal therapeutic care
  (d) Stress and communication

(7) Changing the decision

(8) Objections and challenges
    (a) Challenging the determination of lack of capacity
    (b) Challenging a surrogate
    (c) Futility
    (d) Disagreement on the health care team
    (e) Withdrawal of health care professional or institution

(9) Special comments
    (a) Children
    (b) All invasive procedures included
    (c) Presumption in favor of oral intake
    (d) Need for policy and monitoring
    (e) Education and consultation
    (f) Correcting incentives

PART TWO:
Specific Treatment Modalities

Section C.
GUIDELINES ON MEDICAL PROCEDURES FOR SUPPLYING NUTRITION AND HYDRATION

I. INTRODUCTION

Among the most effective and widely used methods of sustaining life are medical procedures for supplying nutrition and hydration by tubes, catheters, or needles inserted into the patient's body. Forgoing these procedures is controversial and presents a special ethical problem. On the one hand, they provide food and water, which are often regarded as non-medical means of sustaining life that must be provided in all cases. On the other hand, these methods are also artificial (man-made) means of providing care, requiring the efforts of medical personnel and bodily invasion. They impose burdens as well as provide benefits, and therefore can be considered medical interventions which, like other interventions, may under some circumstances be forgone.

We have concluded that it is wisest and most plausible to understand these methods as medical interventions that may be forgone in some cases. Therefore, the standards to be used for decisions concerning termination of these procedures are essentially those that apply for the termination of other forms of medical treatment. At the same time, the issue has only recently received widespread attention. It provokes strong feelings, and for some a sense of moral offense. There is also concern about potential abuse. Thus caution is necessary.

In reaching these conclusions, we have recognized that food and water undeniably have a symbolic and psychological importance. They symbolize our caring for and nurturing of one another, and can be a means for the patient to obtain comfort and satisfaction. In certain circumstances, however, the patient experiences more comfort, caring, and satisfaction from forgoing medical procedures for supplying nutrition and hydration, and instead receiving supportive care to keep him or her comfortable.

Malnutrition and dehydration are conditions determined by chemical tests. They are not the same as the felt states of hunger and thirst. Medical procedures for supplying nutrition and hydration treat malnutrition and dehydration; they may or may not relieve hunger and thirst. Conversely, hunger and thirst can be treated without necessarily using medical nutrition and hydration techniques and without necessarily correcting dehydration or malnourishment. For instance, dehydrated patients may have their thirst relieved by having their lips and mouths moistened with ice chips or lubricant. Moreover, patients in their last days before death may spontaneously reduce their intake of nutrition and hydration without experiencing hunger or thirst. (See BIBLIOGRAPHY.)

Consequently, in some cases medical procedures for supplying nutrition and hydration and the life these procedures offer may impose burdens that exceed their benefits to the patient, or may be contrary to the patient's known wishes. These Guidelines thus reject the contention that medical procedures for supplying nutrition and hydration should automatically be used whenever oral intake is chemically inadequate. Even though they are overwhelmingly beneficial in most situations, these procedures present options that must be evaluated in each case. Time-limited trials are particularly useful in evaluating nutrition and hydration options. Trials of either treatment or forgoing treatment can be used to assess the associated benefits and burdens.

II. GUIDELINES ON MEDICAL PROCEDURES FOR SUPPLYING NUTRITION AND HYDRATION

[REMEMBER: The Guidelines below are amendments and additions to the corresponding sections of PART ONE. They must be read together with PART ONE.]

(2) Evaluation and discussion.

(a) **Evaluating the patient.** Because nutrition and hydration deficits can be subtle and difficult to detect, particularly in seriously ill patients, and because of widespread concern about possible neglect of patients' nutrition and hydration needs in various settings, we recommend procedures that encourage patient evaluations. Whenever the responsible health care professional has reason to suspect that the patient's current means of nutrition and hydration are failing to meet the patient's physiological and psychological needs, the professional should perform an evaluation. The professional should consult with dieticians, nurses, and others with relevant expertise and information. The professional should reevaluate the patient's nutrition and hydration status whenever warranted, and at regular and established intervals. A patient's nutrition and hydration status may change. Difficulty in swallowing, for example, may be intermittent or short-term, allowing oral intake to resume, or a patient's nutrition and hydration status may deteriorate.

(b) **Facilitating discussion.** Discussing the possibility of forgoing medical procedures for supplying nutrition or hydration will often be troubling, and health care personnel will often have understandable resistance to initiating discussion. However, since patients and surrogates frequently give less thought to forgoing nutrition than other forms of life-sustaining treatment, it is especially important to provide opportunities for the patient, surrogate, or others to raise the issue. Introducing the question with open-ended and non-judgmental inquiries may help initiate discussion.

(6) Implementing the decision.

(a) **Time-limited trials.** Time-limited trials of medical procedures for supplying nutrition and hydration are highly recommended. Whether a procedure will be effective and what burdens and benefits it will entail may often be unclear. Time-limited trials of forgoing such medical procedures may also be useful in ascertaining the benefits and burdens.

(b) **Supportive care.** When an ethically appropriate decision has been made to forgo medical procedures for supplying nutrition or hydration, any suffering by the patient should be ameliorated by appropriate treatment, with the patient's or surrogate's consent. A decision to forgo medical procedures for supplying nutrition and hydration does not preclude offering food and fluids for the purpose of physical or psychological comfort.

(9) Special considerations.

(b) **All invasive procedures included.** All invasive procedures for supplying nutrition and hydration—all enteral and parenteral techniques—should be considered procedures that require the patient's or surrogate's consent, and procedures that the patient or surrogate may choose to forgo. This includes not only procedures such as use of a gastrostomy or jejunostomy tube, but also the nasogastric (NG) tube and the peripheral intravenous line (IV). The practice has been not to seek consent for these latter two procedures because they have been considered part of the routine care consented to on admission to the health care institution. However, all medical techniques for supplying nutrition and hydration that involve bodily invasion should be a matter of choice by the patient or surrogate, except when begun on an emergency basis with no time for consent (see PART TWO: Section B on Emergency Interventions); the degree of invasiveness of the procedure should not determine the need for consent. In some cases, an NG tube or IV line will have to be initiated on an emergency basis. If this can be anticipated, consent can be sought before the emergency. If not, the question of whether the patient or surrogate chooses to discontinue this treatment can be confronted after treatment is under way.

(c) Presumption in favor of oral intake. Patients should receive nutrition and hydration orally if possible; in most cases this is better for the patient nutritionally and psychologically. If oral intake does not meet the patient's needs, the responsible health care professional should consult with the patient, and with relevant staff such as dieticians and nurses, to find out what adjustments may improve the adequacy of oral intake. Any reasonable adjustments should be tried. For example, the patient may prefer certain foods. Providing oral nutritional supplements or hand feeding (see GLOSSARY) may also improve the patient's nutritional intake. Oral intake, including hand feeding and oral nutritional supplements, should be offered to all patients capable of it, even if they are also receiving nutrition and hydration by other means. Oral intake should not be forced on a patient. Limits on staff time, numbers, and education as well as reimbursement policies can be barriers to the oral feeding of patients. These and other disincentives to oral feeding should be identified and eliminated to the extent reasonably possible.

(d) Need for policy and monitoring. Because of the controversial nature of decisions to forgo medical procedures for supplying nutrition and hydration and because of the potential for abuse, health care institutions should develop written policy on these decisions. Institutions should also monitor and periodically review decisions made both to forgo and to provide medical procedures for supplying nutrition or hydration.

(e) Education and consultation. There are great differences from institution to institution, and health care professional to health care professional, in the level of expertise on nutrition and hydration needs and options. Professionals have an obligation to educate themselves in this area and obtain appropriate consultations, and institutions should assess their need for in-house educational programs.

(f) Correcting incentives. In some institutions, financial incentives and organizational arrangements make it difficult to adjust a patient's means of nutrition and hydration according to the patient's or surrogate's preferences. These problems are barriers to putting these Guidelines into effect. Institutional administrators and members of the health care team who are aware of these incentives can recommend and undertake systemic changes that will allow the Guidelines to function successfully.

PART TWO:
Specific Treatment Modalities
Section D.
*GUIDELINES ON ANTIBIOTICS AND OTHER
LIFE-SUSTAINING MEDICATION*

I. INTRODUCTION

II. GUIDELINES ON ANTIBIOTICS AND OTHER
LIFE-SUSTAINING MEDICATION

[NOTE: These Guidelines on antibiotics build on PART
ONE. Sections not underlined below are found in PART
ONE and apply here without amendment. Where a section
is underlined, amendments or additions to that section of
PART ONE appear here.]

(1) Underlying ethical values
   (a) <u>Patient well-being—benefiting more than burdening the
       patient</u>
   (b) Patient self-determination
   (c) The ethical integrity of health care professionals
   (d) <u>Justice or equity</u>

(2) Evaluation and discussion
   (a) <u>Evaluating the patient</u>
   (b) <u>Facilitating discussion</u>

(3) Identifying the key decisionmaker
   (a) Assessing decisionmaking capacity
   (b) Identifying a surrogate
   (c) The patient who lacks a ready surrogate

(4) Making the decision
   (a) The patient with decisionmaking capacity
   (b) The patient whose capacity is fluctuating or uncertain
   (c) <u>The patient who lacks decisionmaking capacity</u>

(5) <u>Documenting the decision</u>

(6) Implementing the decision
   (a) Time-limited trials
   (b) <u>Supportive care</u>
   (c) Maximal therapeutic care
   (d) <u>Stress and communication</u>

(7) Changing the decision

(8) Objections and challenges
 (a) Challenging the determination of lack of capacity
 (b) Challenging a surrogate
 (c) Futility
 (d) Disagreement on the health care team
 (d) Withdrawal of health care professional or institution

(9) Special comments
 (a) Children

PART TWO:
Specific Treatment Modalities

Section D.
GUIDELINES ON ANTIBIOTICS AND OTHER
LIFE-SUSTAINING MEDICATION

I. INTRODUCTION

Antibiotics have assumed great importance as one of the revolutionary agents that modern medicine has developed to save lives. They are viewed as "wonder drugs" that can usually be administered simply, safely, and dependably to overcome infections that would otherwise be serious and even life-threatening. It is often assumed that administering antibiotics is invariably beneficial, and that it would be wrong not to provide them to all patients with bacterial infections. As a result, antibiotics are given routinely to nearly all patients with signs of infection. Other life-sustaining medications, such as vasopressors, are also viewed as part of the essential medical armamentarium that health care professionals must employ to treat their patients. Yet the availability of such medication does not resolve the question of whether it should always be used. These Guidelines focus on the ethical issues that the use of antibiotics and other life-sustaining medication raises.

Although many people believe that administering antibiotics is simple and benign, this is not necessarily so. The fact that antibiotics may generally be provided non-invasively and without complex equipment does not resolve the ethical question of whether they ought to be used. Administering these drugs can be burdensome in some respects. Repeated injections and the progressive loss of and increasingly difficult search for suitable injection sites can create considerable pain and suffering for patients. Antibiotics may lead to complications and substantial risk for some patients. Further, giving antibiotics and other antimicrobials in some cases will prolong pain and suffering and ultimately prove futile in fighting infection. Some patients experience a series of increasingly serious and painful reinfections that lead to gradual and severe deterioration of their health.

Although administering these drugs can constitute a beneficial and welcome form of life-sustaining treatment for many patients, for others it can be disproportionately burdensome. Some patients who are terminally ill or in a severely debilitated and irreversible condition may determine that treatment with antibiotics will only prolong their pain and suffering. Decisions about using antibiotics and other life-sustaining medication, like decisions about other forms of life-sustaining treatment, require patients or their surrogates to balance carefully the potential burdens of the treatment and the life it offers against the benefits.

II. GUIDELINES ON ANTIBIOTICS AND OTHER LIFE-SUSTAINING MEDICATION

[REMEMBER: The Guidelines below are amendments and additions to the corresponding sections of PART ONE. They must be read together with PART ONE.]

(1) Underlying ethical values.

(a) **Patient well-being—benefiting more than burdening the patient.** There is a widely held assumption among health care professionals that providing antibiotics is invariably beneficial to the patient. This is not the case. The patient or surrogate should be able to evaluate and forgo antibiotics as they can other forms of treatment.

(d) **Justice or equity.** Overriding a patient's refusal of antibiotics or other life-sustaining medication may be necessary for public health reasons. It may be necessary to administer antibiotics to an unwilling patient with tuberculosis, for instance, to prevent contagion. A patient's wishes, however, should prevail unless there is legal authorization to override those wishes.

(2) Evaluation and discussion.

(a) **Evaluating the patient.** As with other life-sustaining treatments, an evaluation should be done to determine the benefits and burdens of administering antibiotics; the medication should not be given solely as a means of avoiding a decisionmaking process. In order to diagnose the source of an infection or other lesion and evaluate the advisability of antibiotics, health care professionals sometimes consider using invasive procedures or admitting a patient to the hospital. If the patient is likely to suffer disproportionately from such measures, professionals should consider whether those measures can be forgone and treatment decisions made on the basis of a presumptive diagnosis instead.

(b) **Facilitating discussion.** The patient or surrogate should be told how antibiotics or other life-sustaining medication would most likely affect the feasibility of other forms of life-sustaining treatment. In addition, the patient or surrogate should be informed of the means available to relieve painful and distressing symptoms that may occur with or without these drugs.

(4) Making the decision.

(c) The patient who lacks decisionmaking capacity.

1. **Follow the patient's explicit directives.** When the surrogate is choosing in accordance with the patient's explicit directives, the surrogate can derive the patient's preferences about antibiotics or other life-sustaining medication from statements about the use of "general medical care." These statements may appear in an advance directive or other writing (see PART THREE), or as an oral expression of preference. The terms "antibiotics," "antimicrobials," or "life-sustaining medication" need not be used explicitly, since they are considered a form of "general medical care."

2. **Or apply the patient's preferences and values.**

3. **Or choose as a reasonable person in the patient's circumstances would.** A surrogate who applies either the patient's preferences and values or the "reasonable person" standard should consider the patient's overall condition and the potential for clinical improvement, rather than asking only whether the specific infection will respond to treatment.

(5) Documenting the decision.
When antibiotics or other medication would be life-sustaining, a decision to forgo their use should be documented in the patient's medical record.

(6) Implementing the decision.

(b) Supportive care.
Patients who forgo antibiotics or other life-sustaining medication may suffer painful or uncomfortable symptoms of their infection. At the time a decision is made to forgo medication, ways to relieve such foreseeable symptoms should be incorporated into the supportive care plan. Should such symptoms arise unexpectedly after medication has stopped, the responsible health care professional should consider means to relieve them. (See also PART TWO: Section E.)

(d) Stress and communication.
Health care professionals may wonder whether they have fulfilled their obligations to the patient when an untreated infection is aesthetically offensive, for instance because it is gangrenous and malodorous. Such offensiveness

does not make the decision to forgo the administration of life-sustaining medication unethical. Health care professionals should explore ways to improve the situation for all. In rare circumstances, a severely offensive situation may be so distressing that the patient may have to accept treatments that make care possible in order to stay in that health care institution.

PART TWO:
Specific Treatment Modalities

Section E.
GUIDELINES ON PALLIATIVE CARE AND THE RELIEF OF PAIN

I. INTRODUCTION

II. GUIDELINES ON PALLIATIVE CARE AND THE RELIEF OF PAIN

[Note: These Guidelines on palliative care build on PART ONE. Sections not underlined below are found in PART ONE and apply here without amendment. Where a section is underlined, amendments or additions to that section of PART ONE appear here.]

(1) Underlying ethical values
    (a) Patient well-being—benefiting more than burdening the patient
    (b) Patient self-determination
    (c) The ethical integrity of health care professionals
    (d) Justice or equity

(2) Evaluation and discussion
    (a) Evaluating the patient
    (b) Facilitating discussion

(3) Identifying the key decisionmaker
    (a) Assessing decisionmaking capacity
    (b) Identifying a surrogate
    (c) The patient who lacks a ready surrogate

(4) Making the decision
    (a) The patient with decisionmaking capacity
    (b) The patient whose capacity is fluctuating or uncertain
    (c) The patient who lacks decisionmaking capacity

(5) Documenting the decision

(6) Implementing the decision
    (a) Time-limited trials
    (b) Supportive care
    (c) Maximal therapeutic care
    (d) Stress and communication

(7) Changing the decision

(8) Objections and challenges
    (a) Challenging the determination of lack of capacity
    (b) Challenging a surrogate
    (c) Futility
    (d) Disagreement on the health care team
    (e) Withdrawal of health care professional or institution

(9) Special comments
    (a) Children
    (b) Developing a plan for palliative care and pain relief
    (c) Funding and incentives

PART TWO:
Specific Treatment Modalities

Section E.
*GUIDELINES ON PALLIATIVE CARE AND THE
RELIEF OF PAIN*

I. INTRODUCTION

Patients who are dying can experience many different symptoms, such as acute and chronic pain, dyspnea, and nausea. The primary goals of treatment, unless the patient chooses otherwise, are to relieve pain and suffering and to help the patient function as fully as possible. Health care professionals have an obligation to control distressing symptoms in dying patients. The suffering of these patients can result not only from physical causes, but from emotional, social, and spiritual ones as well. Their total care requires professionals to pay attention to all these potential origins of distress.

Patients usually want palliative care and pain relief, and health care professionals have an obligation to provide both. Sometimes, however, patients or surrogates wish to forgo such treatment, to maintain alertness, for example. Although the decisionmaking process in PART ONE concerns forgoing treatment that is life-sustaining rather than palliative, it is a basic format that can also be used for making decisions about palliative care and pain relief, with the modifications suggested below.

Palliative care refers generically to medical, surgical, and other procedures that are used to alleviate suffering, discomfort, and dysfunction. Palliative care can include efforts such as surgery, radiation, chemotherapy, or the administration of antibiotics, if any of these will make the patient more comfortable. For some patients, by contrast, distressing symptoms can be alleviated only by ending therapeutic efforts such as chemotherapy or ventilator use. A patient's particular situation must be carefully considered in striving for symptomatic relief and improved functioning; patients differ tremendously in their evaluations of the experiences associated with dying and the degree of function that they wish to maintain. No single mode of palliative care will be appropriate for all patients with similar symptoms. However, all dying patients should be assured that professionals will listen attentively to them and provide emotional reassurance, physical contact, and social support.

Pain relief refers specifically to measures to alleviate pain. Although the majority of dying patients do not feel substantial pain, most fear the possibility of pain—perhaps more than death itself. The anxiety of these patients can be mitigated by developing with them a plan for pain relief and palliative care and by a confident and reassuring approach. Since the primary goal of caring for dying patients is to relieve pain and suffering unless the patient or surrogate chooses otherwise, measures involving substantial risk may be considered (such as destroying certain nerves by injecting drugs), although they might not be undertaken to relieve the discomfort of patients with a reasonable chance for survival.

Drugs may also be administered to alleviate pain for patients who are dying. Unfortunately, health care professionals currently tend to provide narcotic agents in insufficient amounts to prevent or relieve pain for these patients. Many health care professionals have inadequate knowledge about the pharmacology of pain relief and the appropriate use of narcotics and similar agents for dying patients. Moreover, even those who are knowledgeable do not always agree about appropriate dosages for individual patients. As a result, some patients near death do not receive adequate pain medication, and end their lives in great suffering. There is a pressing need to develop and disseminate more adequate information about the use of narcotics and other methods of pain relief.

Health care professionals and families are also sometimes concerned that dying patients may become addicted to narcotics, and professionals consequently tend to provide insufficient doses. This concern arises from a confusion between physical and psychological dependence, and from a misunderstanding of the dangers each poses for dying patients. People who are physically dependent experience distressing symptoms of withdrawal if narcotics are suddenly withdrawn. People who are psychologically dependent desire drugs and become driven to obtain them. In dying patients physical dependence regularly occurs but psychological dependence is rare. Physical dependence does not trouble patients who are dying, for the administration of narcotics need never end abruptly and cause them distress. Psychological dependence is uncommon but can create greater difficulties. However, psychological dependence often results from under- rather than overmedication; patients are less likely to become psychologically dependent when narcotic agents are given on a prophylactic schedule, rather than in response to a request after pain is experienced. Since psychological dependence is rare, health care professionals should address the problem on those few occasions when it occurs rather than allowing the majority of dying patients to suffer out of a misplaced fear of psychological dependence.

Finally, there is a belief that providing narcotics to dying patients might constitute a form of wrongful killing, since it can lead to respiratory depression and hasten death. Providing large quantities of narcotic analgesics does not constitute wrongful killing when the purpose is not to shorten the lives of these patients, but to alleviate their pain and suffering, and the alternatives have been carefully evaluated and this course found to serve the patient best. Sometimes the degree of suffering that dying patients experience is sufficiently severe to warrant risking an earlier death. Further, there is some evidence that administering narcotic agents in amounts sufficient to provide adequate pain relief may extend, rather than shorten, life. This is because patients without pain are more likely to accept a greater degree of nourishment, to be more active and less depressed, and to be more open to other treatment possibilities. As a result, they may live longer. There are no sound moral grounds for failing to provide adequate relief from pain to those who are dying and wish such relief.

Patients occasionally ask for medication in order to commit suicide. This raises a substantial ethical problem on which there is societal disagreement, and which is beyond the scope of these Guidelines. (See PART SIX: Section I.)

II. GUIDELINES ON PALLIATIVE CARE AND THE RELIEF OF PAIN

[REMEMBER: The Guidelines below are amendments and additions to the corresponding sections of PART ONE. They must be read together with PART ONE.]

(1) Underlying ethical values.

(a) **Patient well-being—benefiting more than burdening the patient.** Once a decision has been made to forgo life-sustaining treatment and death is expected to ensue, the primary benefit that professionals can provide is usually relief from pain and suffering and enhancement of the patient's opportunity for satisfying experiences.

(b) **Patient self-determination.** Since patients know most fully the extent of their suffering and their need for relief, their wishes about palliative care and pain relief should guide professionals. Whenever possible, the patient together with the responsible health care professional should determine the degree and type of palliation and pain relief. When the patient cannot do so, the surrogate should make that determination with the professional. (See Section (4) (c), p. 74.)

Adequate palliation and pain relief do not ordinarily impair the patient's decisionmaking capacity. Sometimes, however, relief of pain and suffering will produce impairment. Whenever possible, the patient should decide what level of relief and decisionmaking capacity he or she prefers. When sedation is likely to reduce the patient's decisionmaking capacity, the health care professional should try to secure clear advance directions from the patient about the content of future care.

(c) The ethical integrity of health care professionals. Health care professionals have an obligation to affirm the values of compassion and humanity by mitigating the pain and suffering of the dying. They have a responsibility to be technically competent in palliation and pain relief and to provide adequate symptom control.

Some health care professionals worry that administering large quantities of pain-relieving drugs to dying patients constitutes professional incompetence. To the contrary, the primary goal in caring for the dying (unless the patient or surrogate chooses otherwise) is to mitigate pain and suffering; thus the health care professional who does so is acting in accord with the fundamental professional requirement to promote the patient's good.

(2) Evaluation and discussion.

(a) Evaluating the patient. Treating the patient with pain-relieving drugs may be necessary to improve his or her ability to participate in this evaluation and to develop a plan for palliative care and pain relief. Reevaluation of the patient's response to prescribed therapy must be frequent, since patients' needs for palliation and pain relief change over time.

(4) Making the decision.

(a) The patient with decisionmaking capacity. Some patients with decisionmaking capacity may elect not to have all available palliative care and pain relief administered to them, sometimes in order to remain alert. The patient's wishes concerning the amount of pain relief and palliative care should control.

(c) The patient who lacks decisionmaking capacity. A surrogate's decision to forgo palliative care and the relief of pain can sometimes lead to a painful death for a patient without decisionmaking capacity. If that seems likely, the decision should be subject to review by the institutional ethics committee or other institutional mechanism for advising on ethical issues.

(5) Documenting the decision. An order for the use of pain-killing agents and palliative treatment requires careful documentation in order to ensure continuity of care. The order should clearly state why the drug dosages were prescribed, and should indicate their purpose. When a patient with decisionmaking capacity decides to forgo palliative care and pain-relieving drugs, this should be documented in the patient's records so that other involved health care professionals will be informed.

(6) Implementing the decision.

(b) Supportive care. Palliative care and pain relief are central components of supportive care. It is important to attempt to relieve all forms of suffering and pain (unless the patient or surrogate chooses otherwise), whether the patient is forgoing or receiving a life-sustaining treatment. When the patient or surrogate elects to forgo palliative care and pain relief, the patient should nonetheless receive whatever supportive care is consistent with that choice. (See also Section (4) (c), p. 74.)

(9) Special comments.

(b) Developing a plan for palliative care and pain relief. The responsible health care professional should inform the patient or surrogate about the forms of palliative care and pain relief that are available. Together they should formulate a plan for palliative care and pain relief. The plan should encompass not only current measures, but also future measures to be taken if the patient's circumstances change.

(c) Funding and incentives. Inadequate reimbursement and funding for appropriate palliative care and pain relief, and a lack of organized provider agencies, are substantial problems. Effective palliative care and pain relief are part of minimally adequate health care. Thus, public and private insurers, state health planning agencies, quality assurance programs, regulators of provider agencies, and educators should seek to ensure that effective palliative care and pain relief are available to patients, including those forgoing all other treatment. Health care professionals should resist financial and organizational incentives that discourage adequate palliative care and pain relief.

PART THREE:
Prospective Planning
GUIDELINES ON ADVANCE DIRECTIVES

I. INTRODUCTION

II. GENERAL GUIDELINES ON ADVANCE DIRECTIVES

(1) Definitions
    (a) Treatment directive
    (b) Proxy directive

(2) Developing a directive

(3) Proof of execution

(4) Implementation
    (a) Notice to the responsible health care professional
    (b) Communication to surrogate(s), family, and concerned friends
    (c) Presentation on admission to a health care institution

(5) Review and revision

(6) Revocation

III. ADDITIONAL GUIDELINES ON TREATMENT DIRECTIVES INCLUDING "LIVING WILLS"

(1) Components
    (a) Present decisionmaking capacity
    (b) General treatment preferences
    (c) Use of specific treatments
    (d) Use of palliative care and pain relief
    (e) Treatment setting
    (f) Surrogate appointment
    (g) Other statements
    (h) Attachment of treatment plan

IV. ADDITIONAL GUIDELINES ON PROXY DIRECTIVES

(1) Components

(a) Consent to and refusal of treatment
(b) Legal releases
(c) Changing health care professionals and health care institutions
(d) Access to medical records
(e) Court authorization for treatment decisions

(2) Alternate surrogates

(3) Effect of proxy directive

PART THREE:
Prospective Planning
GUIDELINES ON ADVANCE DIRECTIVES

I. INTRODUCTION

One of the major goals of these Guidelines is to encourage patients and their health care professionals to plan about treatment in advance of a crisis, and while the patient still has decisionmaking capacity. When the patient is diagnosed as having a condition that may eventually raise questions about the termination of treatment, the responsible health care professional and patient should begin talking about future options as early as possible.

In some cases, the responsible health care professional may feel it would be useful to write a formal treatment plan; more often the planning process will take place in a series of discussions between the patient and professional, with notations made in the patient's records. The planning process has several purposes: to develop a rapport between the patient and the health care professional; to identify the patient's preferences, values, and priorities that bear on future treatment decisions, particularly concerning life-sustaining treatment; and to help ensure consistent treatment for the patient as he or she comes under the care of different health care professionals in various institutional settings. Sometimes a patient will want to augment this planning process by writing an advance directive.

An advance directive is a document allowing a person to give directions about future medical care, or to designate who should make medical decisions if he or she should lose decisionmaking capacity. There are two types of advance directives. In a *treatment directive,* such as a "living will," a person can indicate those treatments, including life-sustaining treatment, in particular, that the person wishes to receive or forgo should he or she be in stated medical conditions (such as irreversible unconsciousness, severe and irreversible dementia, or terminal illness) and lack decisionmaking capacity. In that document, or in a separate *proxy directive,* a person can identify a surrogate to make treatment decisions should he or she be unable to make such decisions.

The following Guidelines provide assistance to individuals who wish to develop advance directives and to professionals counseling individuals. This Section of the Guidelines refers to legal requirements to a greater extent than any other. This is because when an advance directive deviates from the requirements of the relevant statute or when no state law authorizes advance directives, the directive might not be regarded as legally effective and might not be followed. To guard against this, a patient should consult with a lawyer if possible, and discuss the advance directive thoroughly with health care professionals, family, and concerned friends.

Treatment directives have been recognized by statute in most states and the District of Columbia. The statutes authorizing them differ considerably in their terms. Many apply only to persons who formerly had decisionmaking capacity and who will die imminently with or without life-sustaining treatment. Thus, they cover a very narrow range of cases, and assist only persons who are on the verge of death. Treatment directives have also been recognized in judicial decisions, in cases not covered by statute.

Proxy directives have been recognized in a number of states in different kinds of legislation, including various durable power of attorney (DPA) statutes (see GLOSSARY) allowing the appointment of a proxy decisionmaker, and some statutes that authorize both treatment directives and proxy directives. We suggest that all jurisdictions adopt statutes permitting the use of a DPA to designate a surrogate for health care decisionmaking.

Some states require a precise format for advance directives; individuals should follow this format whenever possible to maximize the likelihood that the directive will be followed, and then add further instructions if they wish. Other state statutes allow deviation from the form recommended in the statute. In states with no statute authorizing advance directives there is no form to follow. Despite the lack of a statute, advance directives may still have legal effect as an exercise of the patient's right to decide about treatment.

A directive that is legally effective in the state where it was drawn up may not have formal statutory recognition in the state where the patient receives treatment. A few states have provided in their statutes for the recognition of directives executed out of state. We recommend that health care professionals honor an out-of-state directive as an expression of the individual's wishes.

This Section bears a close relationship to PART ONE, the basic decisionmaking section. This Section concerns the development of advance directives; PART ONE addresses using those directives in making treatment decisions. Ideally, a patient would first go through a planning process and draw up advance directives, and later the patient or the patient's surrogate would make treatment decisions as recommended in PART ONE, building on the planning process and directives. As we state in PART ONE, health care professionals and surrogates should honor advance directives.

II. GENERAL GUIDELINES ON ADVANCE DIRECTIVES

These Guidelines apply to both treatment directives and proxy directives.

(1) Definitions.

(a) A **treatment directive** is a written statement prepared by an individual directing which forms of medical treatment the individual wishes to receive or forgo should he or she be in stated medical conditions (such as irreversible unconsciousness, severe and irreversible dementia, or terminal illness) and lack decisionmaking capacity. A "living will" is a type of treatment directive.

(b) A **proxy directive** is a written statement in which an individual appoints another person to make his or her health care decisions in the event that the designating individual lacks the capacity to do so. A proxy directive may appear as part of a treatment directive or it may be a separate document.

A common form that proxy directives take, but not the only form, is a durable power of attorney (DPA). A DPA is a written designation in which an individual names a person (*i.e.,* a surrogate) to act on his or her behalf in the event that he or she loses decisionmaking capacity. A durable power of attorney differs from a power of attorney in that the latter authorization terminates when the designating individual loses decisionmaking capacity, whereas the former does not.

(2) Developing a directive. Adults with decisionmaking capacity should prepare advance directives. Some minors may also wish to develop treatment directives, which should be considered by health care professionals and honored whenever possible. (See PART ONE: Section (9), p. 33.)

The responsible health care professional should discuss advance directives with the patient as early as possible. Health care institutions should facilitate the development of such directives. Attorneys should educate themselves about advance directives and discuss them with clients as a part of estate planning.

(3) **Proof of execution.** State law should be followed in executing the directive. In any case, the directive should be signed by the individual and dated.

(4) **Implementation.** Relevant persons should be informed of the existence and contents of the directive.

(a) **Notice to the responsible health care professional.** The individual should discuss the directive with the health care professional responsible for his or her care. The individual should ask that copies be filed in the medical record in the professional's office. If the responsible health care professional is unwilling to comply with a directive, the patient should consider changing caregivers.

(b) **Communication to surrogate(s), family, and concerned friends.** The individual should also inform the designated surrogate and alternate surrogates (if any), family members, and concerned friends of the existence of any directives, and should give them copies as seems appropriate.

(c) **Presentation on admission to a health care institution.** When an individual is admitted to a health care institution, the admitting health care professional should determine whether the patient has an advance directive. If so, copies of the directive should be entered into the medical record, and a notation made in the record of its existence.

(5) **Review and revision.** The individual should review the directive every one or two years to ensure that it continues to represent his or her wishes. The individual may make additions, changes, and deletions at any time. State law should be followed in making changes. In the absence of state law requirements, changes should be clearly initialed, dated, and witnessed. These changes should also be made in copies that have been distributed to health care professionals, surrogates, family members, and others.

(6) **Revocation.** The individual may revoke either a treatment or proxy directive at any time, either orally or in writing. Notice of revocation should be given to the designated surrogate or surrogates, if any. Pertinent state law, if any, should be consulted on the recommended means of revocation. Notice of revocation should be given to those who have received copies of the directive.

III. ADDITIONAL GUIDELINES ON TREATMENT DIRECTIVES INCLUDING "LIVING WILLS"

(1) **Components.** When state statutes provide for treatment directives, those statutes should be consulted. The following components are recommended for treatment directives:

(a) **Present decisionmaking capacity.** The directive should contain a declaration of the individual's present capacity to make decisions and a statement that the individual is acting of his or her own free will.

(b) **General treatment preferences.** The directive should contain a statement about the general preferences of the individual concerning the goals of medical treatment, should the individual be in stated medical conditions and lack decisionmaking capacity.

(c) **Use of specific treatments.** The directive should indicate the preferences of the individual regarding the use of specific kinds of treatments, such as the ventilator, dialysis, cardiopulmonary resuscitation, medical procedures for supplying nutrition and hydration, and antibiotics, should the person be in stated medical conditions and lack decisionmaking capacity.

(d) **Use of palliative care and pain relief.** The directive may contain a statement about the kinds of palliative care and pain relief, in addition to basic hygienic and nursing care, requested by the individual under stated circumstances. For example, a person might authorize medication to the point of unconsciousness if necessary to relieve pain.

(e) **Treatment setting.** The directive may indicate the individual's preferences for home, nursing home, hospital, or hospice care under stated conditions.

(f) **Surrogate appointment.** The directive may contain a statement appointing another person (*i.e.,* a surrogate) to make health care decisions, should the designating individual lack decisionmaking capacity. (See Section IV immediately below.)

(g) **Other statements.** The directive may also include any other matters of importance to the individual, such as the names of persons to whom health care professionals and surrogates can turn for guidance.

(h) **Attachment of treatment plan.** An individual may attach to a substantive directive any written treatment plan that he or she has developed with a health care professional.

IV. ADDITIONAL GUIDELINES ON PROXY DIRECTIVES

(1) **Components.** When state statutes provide for proxy directives, it is important to develop a proxy directive that follows state law. An individual developing a proxy directive may authorize a surrogate to make decisions in any or all of the following areas (subject to state law restrictions) in the event that the designating individual lacks decisionmaking capacity:

(a) **Consent to and refusal of treatment.** The individual may authorize the surrogate to consent to or refuse specific treatments including life-sustaining treatments, palliative care, and pain relief measures.

(b) **Legal releases.** The individual may authorize the surrogate to grant releases from legal liability to health care personnel.

(c) **Changing health care professionals and health care institutions.** The individual may authorize the surrogate to engage and to discharge health care professionals and to admit or remove the individual from health care institutions.

(d) **Access to medical records.** The individual may grant the surrogate access to medical records and other personal information and may permit the surrogate to release such information as needed.

(e) **Court authorization for treatment decisions.** The individual may instruct the surrogate to resort to the courts, if necessary, to obtain authorization regarding medical treatment decisions.

(2) **Choice of surrogate.** Acting as a surrogate is a weighty responsibility. It is important to designate someone who is likely to be able to play this role, willing to do it, and knowledgeable about the designating individual's preferences and values. Before designating someone, the individual should discuss with that person whether he or she feels able and willing to act as surrogate.

(3) **Alternate surrogates.** An individual may designate alternate surrogates. In this event, the individual's choices should be listed in order of priority, and the conditions of succession should be stated (for example, the prior person is unable or unwilling to serve in this role). The individual should discuss with the alternate

surrogates also whether they feel able and willing to take on this responsibility.

(4) **Effect of proxy directive.** If the designating individual loses decisionmaking capacity, health care professionals should notify the surrogate designated by the individual in the proxy directive.

PART FOUR:
Declaring Death
GUIDELINES ON THE DECLARATION OF DEATH

I. INTRODUCTION

II. PROCEDURAL GUIDELINES

(1) Triggering a neurological evaluation

(2) Obligation to declare the patient dead

(3) Cessation of treatment after a declaration of death

(4) Health care professionals who should not make the declaration

APPENDIX: The Report of the Consultants

PART FOUR:
Declaring Death
GUIDELINES ON THE DECLARATION OF DEATH

I. INTRODUCTION

There are two well-established ways to determine reliably that death has occurred: (a) use of cardiopulmonary criteria to assess whether circulatory and respiratory functions have irreversibly ceased, or (b) use of neurological criteria to assess whether all brain functions have irreversibly ceased when cardiopulmonary functions are maintained artificially.

Most states now recognize, through statutes or judicial decisions, that death may be determined on the basis of neurological criteria. In the remaining states the law has not yet explicitly departed from the older, common-law view that death occurs when cardiopulmonary functions have ceased.

Agreement is now widespread that when there has been irreversible loss of cardiopulmonary functions or of all brain functions, death should be declared. Many prominent groups have endorsed the following model statute:

Uniform Determination Of Death Act

An individual who has sustained either (1) irreversible cessation of circulatory and respiratory functions, or (2) irreversible cessation of all functions of the entire brain, including the brain stem, is dead. A determination of death must be made in accordance with accepted medical standards.

(See LIST OF SELECTED LEGAL AUTHORITIES.)

These Guidelines adopt the formulation of the model statute and we strongly urge its adoption in all states that have not yet done so. Both the Guidelines and model statute require cessation of the functions of the entire brain (whole brain death) rather than merely the higher brain (neocortical death) or a persistent vegetative state as the basis for determining death. A broad consensus has developed that, regardless of the conflicting religious and secular perspectives on what death is, as a policy matter death should be declared applying whole brain death criteria rather than these alternative criteria that would encompass more patients. The law of all states that have adopted neurological criteria for the declaration of death has accepted this view.

The model statute refers to "accepted medical standards." The medical standards used for determining whether the neurological criteria are met will change with medical developments. The health care professional should make the determination of death in accordance with reasonable standards of medical practice at the time of the assessment. The medical consultants to the President's Commission for the Study of Ethical Problems in Medicine and Biomedical and Behavioral Research set forth accepted medical standards in Appendix F to the report of the President's Commission entitled *Defining Death.* (See BIBLIOGRAPHY.) Their report, referred to here as the *Report of the Consultants,* is reprinted as an Appendix to this Part of the Guidelines.

Those states that have not yet formally adopted neurological criteria for the declaration of death pose special problems for health care professionals. Because the neurological criteria have been so widely accepted, some advocate that health care professionals use the same standards even in states that have not yet formally adopted them. In Section (2), p. 88, we recommend some steps that the health care professional can take in a state that fails to recognize neurological criteria.

Although there is widespread agreement on the use of neurological criteria, the agreement is not universal. In particular, some religious groups, including Orthodox Jews, object. Religious freedom and pluralism are important values in our society. However, in many areas society is forced to have consistent standards. We believe that the societal need for consistency and clarity in determining death mandates as much uniformity as possible in the criteria for declaring death. (See PART SIX: Section VI.) Accordingly, when a patient meets the neurological criteria, the Guidelines do not leave a declaration of death to the discretion of the health care professional, surrogate, family, or others.

Unlike the sections of PART TWO, which concern decisions about various treatment modalities, the Guidelines on the declaration of death *do not* build on the Guidelines on the Decisionmaking Process in PART ONE. Those basic decisionmaking Guidelines are founded on a decisionmaking partnership between the health care professional and the patient or surrogate; the patient or surrogate consents to or refuses treatment. This framework does not apply to death, though there is much remaining confusion on this point in clinical settings. A determination of death is neither chosen nor rejected; it depends only on the patient's physiological state. Consequently, the Guidelines that follow stand independently of PART ONE.

II. PROCEDURAL GUIDELINES FOR THE DECLARATION OF DEATH

These procedural Guidelines are intended to augment the *Report of the Consultants* set forth in the Appendix to this Part.

(1) **Triggering a neurological evaluation.** As soon as the responsible health care professional has a reasonable suspicion that an irreversible loss of all brain functions has occurred, he or she should perform the appropriate tests and procedures to determine the patient's neurological status. This is intended, in part, to avoid the practice of evaluating only those patients who have been identified as potential organ donors. That practice creates a mistaken link between the declaration of death by neurological criteria and organ donation. It has also meant that some patients who are dead by neurological criteria are not declared dead and continue to receive treatment. This perpetuates the common misconception that a patient who is dead by neurological criteria is somehow less dead than a patient who is dead by cardiopulmonary criteria.

(2) **Obligation to declare a patient dead.** Cardiopulmonary criteria for determining death are recognized in all states; when the health care professional determines that the patient has experienced an irreversible cessation of cardiopulmonary functions he or she should declare the patient dead. In most states, the declaration of death based on neurological criteria is also recognized, either by statute or case law. In these states, the patient who has been determined to be dead should promptly be declared dead. Consent of the surrogate, family, or concerned friends is not required. However, the professional should be sensitive to the needs of these people in informing them and providing support. In appropriate circumstances this should include allowing them to obtain a second opinion.

In states where the law does not yet recognize neurological criteria for the declaration of death the proper course of behavior is more uncertain. The health care professional should consult the policy of the health care institution and legal counsel on whether neurological criteria can be used. If the conclusion is that neurological criteria cannot be used as a basis for determining death, the health care professional should at least document the neurological status and inform the patient's surrogate, family, and concerned friends.

Some contend that neurological criteria are now so widely accepted that the professional in a state without law recognizing neurological criteria should behave exactly as would a professional in a state with such law. Others contend that the patient should not be considered dead and choices should be made regarding life-sustaining treatment, in accord with the Guidelines in PARTS ONE and TWO above. This controversy may become moot in the not too distant future if all jurisdictions adopt neurological criteria for determining death. In the meantime, the Guidelines do not advocate acting contrary to legal requirements, but caution health care professionals to ascertain carefully the state of the law and practice in their jurisdiction.

(3) Cessation of treatment after a declaration of death. Once a health care professional has made a declaration of death, all treatment of the patient should ordinarily cease. In some cases the continuation of treatment will be considered because:

(a) efforts are being made to use the patient's body or body parts for any of the purposes stated in the Uniform Anatomical Gift Act (see LIST OF SELECTED LEGAL AUTHORITIES), namely, education, research, advancement of medical or dental science, therapy, and transplantation; or

(b) the patient is pregnant and efforts are being made to save the life of the fetus.

Except for relatively short delays necessary to secure consent, continuing treatment for the above reasons requires appropriate consent and may also require judicial involvement.

Some people contend that if the responsible health care professional is willing, it should be permissible to continue treatment at the family's request (probably for religious reasons) to sustain physiological function in a person who has been determined to be dead by neurological criteria, but whose circulatory and other physiological functions can be sustained. Others—probably most—feel this would be wasteful care or offensive to health care professionals and should not be condoned. At the least, a health care institution that chooses to allow this option should solicit a range of views on the issues raised and adopt explicit policy.

(4) Health care professionals who should not make the declaration. The health care professional who makes the declaration of death should:

(a) not be a member of the organ transplant team, if any, planning or seeking to remove the patient's organs;

(b) not be a member of the patient's family;

(c) not have malpractice charges pending against him or her related to the patient's case; and

(d) not have any other special interest in the declaration of the patient's death, such as standing to inherit under the patient's will.

APPENDIX: The Report of the Consultants

This Appendix reprints Appendix F from the report of the President's Commission for the Study of Ethical Problems in Medicine and Biomedical and Behavioral Research entitled *Defining Death: Medical, Legal and Ethical Issues in the Determination of Death*, Washington, DC: U.S. Government Printing Office, 1981.

GUIDELINES FOR THE DETERMINATION OF DEATH

Report of the Medical Consultants on the Diagnosis of Death to the President's Commission for the Study of Ethical Problems in Medicine and Biomedical and Behavioral Research*

Foreword

The advent of effective artificial cardiopulmonary support for severely brain-injured persons has created some confusion during the past several decades about the determination of death. Previously, loss of heart and lung functions was an easily observable and sufficient basis for diagnosing death, whether the initial failure occurred in the brain, the heart and lungs, or elsewhere in the body. Irreversible failure of either the heart and lungs or the brain precluded the continued functioning of the other. Now, however, circulation and respiration can be maintained by means of a mechanical respirator and other medical interventions, despite a loss of all brain functions. In these circumstances we recognize

---

*The guidelines set forth in this report represent the views of the signatories as individuals; they do not necessarily reflect the policy of any institution or professional association with which any signatory is affiliated. Although the practice of individual signatories may vary slightly, signatories agree on the acceptability of these guidelines: Jesse Barber, M.D., Don Becker, M.D., Richard Behrman, M.D., J.D., Donald R. Bennett, M.D., Richard Beresford, M.D., J.D., Reginald Bickford, M.D., William A. Black, M.D., Benjamin Boshes, M.D., Ph.D., Philip Braunstein, M.D., John Burroughs, M.D., J.D., Russell Butler, M.D., John Caronna, M.D., Shelley Chou, M.D., Ph.D., Kemp Clark, M.D., Ronald Cranford, M.D., Michael Earnest, M.D., Albert Ehle, M.D., Jack M. Fein, M.D., Sal Fiscina, M.D., J.D., Terrance G. Furlow, M.D., J.D., Eli Goldensohn, M.D., Jack Grabow, M.D., Phillip M. Green, M.D., Ake Grenvik, M.D., Charles E. Henry, Ph.D., John Hughes, M.D., Ph.D., D.M., Howard Kaufman, M.D., Robert King, M.D., Julius Korein, M.D., Thomas W. Langfitt, M.D., Cesare Lombroso, M.D., Kevin M McIntyre, M.D., J.D., Richard L. Masland, M.D., Don Harper Mills, M.D., J.D., Gaetano Molinari, M.D., Byron C. Pevehouse, M.D., Lawrence H. Pitts, M.D., A Bernard Pleet, M.D., Fred Plum, M.D., Jerome Posner, M.D., David Powner, M.D., Richard Rovit, M.D., Peter Safar, M.D., Henry Schwartz, M.D., Edward Schlesinger, M.D., Roy Selby, M.D., James Snyer, M.D., Bruce F. Sorenson, M.D., Cary Suter, M.D., Barry Tharp, M.D., Fernando Torres, M.D., A. Earl Walker, M.D., Arthur Ward, M.D., Jack Whisnant, M.D., Robert Wilkus, M.D. and Harry Zimmerman, M.D. The preparation of this report was facilitated by the President's Commission but the guidelines have not been passed on by the Commission and are not intended as matters for governmental review or adoption.

as dead an individual whose loss of brain functions is complete and irreversible.

To recognize reliably that death has occurred, accurate criteria must be available for physicians' use. These now fall into two groups, to be applied depending on the clinical situation. When respiration and circulation have irreversibly ceased, there is no need to assess brain functions directly. When cardiopulmonary functions are artificially maintained, neurologic criteria must be used to assess whether brain functions have irreversibly ceased.

More than half of the states now recognize, through statutes or judicial decisions, that death may be determined on the basis of irreversible cessation of all functions of the brain. Law in the remaining states has not yet departed from the older, common law view that death has not occurred until "all vital functions" (whether or not artificially maintained) have ceased. The language of the statutes has not been uniform from state to state, and the diversity of proposed and enacted laws has created substantial confusion. Consequently, the American Bar Association, the American Medical Association, the National Conference of Commissioners on Uniform State Laws, and the President's Commission for the Study of Ethical Problems in Medicine and Biomedical and Behavioral Research have proposed the following model statute, intended for adoption in every jurisdiction:

Uniform Determination of Death Act
An individual who has sustained either (1) irreversible cessation of circulatory and respiratory functions, or (2) irreversible cessation of all functions of the entire brain, including the brain stem, is dead. A determination of death must be made in accordance with accepted medical standards.

This wording has also been endorsed by the American Academy of Neurology and the American Electroencephalographic Society.

The statute relies upon the existence of "accepted medical standards" for determining that death has occurred. The medical profession, based upon carefully conducted research and extensive clinical experience, has found that death can be reliably determined by either cardiopulmonary or neurologic criteria. The tests used for determining cessation of brain functions have changed and will continue to do so with the advent of new research and technologies. The "Harvard criteria" (JAMA, 205:337, 1968) are widely accepted, but advances in recent years have led to the proposal of other criteria. As an aid to the implementation of the proposed uniform statute, we provide here one statement of currently accepted medical standards.

Introduction

The criteria that physicians use in determining that death has occurred should:

(1) Eliminate errors in classifying a living individual as dead,

(2) Allow as few errors as possible in classifying a dead body as alive,

(3) Allow a determination to be made without unreasonable delay,

(4) Be adaptable to a variety of clinical situations, and

(5) Be explicit and accessible to verification.

Because it would be undesirable for any guidelines to be mandated by legislation or regulation or to be inflexibly established in case law, the proposed Uniform Determination of Death Act appropriately specifies only "accepted medical standards." Local, state, and national institutions and professional organizations are encouraged to examine and publish their practices.

The following guidelines represent a distillation of current practice in regard to the determination of death. Only the most commonly available and verified tests have been included. The time of death recorded on a death certificate is at present a matter of local practice and is not covered in this document.

These guidelines are advisory. Their successful use requires a competent and judicious physician, experienced in clinical examination and the relevant procedures. All periods of observation listed in these guidelines require the patient to be under the care of a physician. Considering the responsibility entailed in the determination of death, consultation is recommended when appropriate.

The outline of the criteria is set forth below in capital letters. The indented text that follows each outline heading explains its meaning. In addition, the two sets of criteria (cardiopulmonary and neurologic) are followed by a presentation of the major complicating conditions: drug and metabolic intoxication, hypothermia, young age, and shock. It is of paramount importance that anyone referring to these guidelines be thoroughly familiar with the entire document, including explanatory notes and complicating conditions.

The Criteria for Determination of Death

An individual presenting the findings in either section A (cardiopulmonary) or section B (neurologic) is dead. In either section, a diagnosis of death requires that *both cessation of functions*, as set forth in subsection 1, *and irreversibility*, as set forth in subsection 2, be demonstrated.

A. AN INDIVIDUAL WITH IRREVERSIBLE CESSATION OF CIRCULATORY AND RESPIRATORY FUNCTIONS IS DEAD.

  1. *CESSATION* IS RECOGNIZED BY AN APPROPRIATE CLINICAL EXAMINATION.
  Clinical examination will disclose at least the absence of responsiveness, heartbeat, and respiratory effort. Medical circumstances may require the use of confirmatory tests, such as an ECG.

  2. *IRREVERSIBILITY* IS RECOGNIZED BY PERSISTENT CESSATION OF FUNCTIONS DURING AN APPROPRIATE PERIOD OF OBSERVATION AND/OR TRIAL OF THERAPY.
  In clinical situations where death is expected, where the course has been gradual, and where irregular agonal respiration or heartbeat finally ceases, the period of observation following the cessation may be only the few minutes required to complete the examination. Similarly, if resuscitation is not undertaken and ventricular fibrillation and standstill develop in a monitored patient, the required period of observation thereafter may be as short as a few minutes. When a possible death is unobserved, unexpected, or sudden, the examination may need to be more detailed and repeated over a longer period, while appropriate resuscitative effort is maintained as a test of cardiovascular responsiveness. Diagnosis in individuals who are first observed with rigor mortis or putrefaction may require only the observation period necessary to establish that fact.

B. AN INDIVIDUAL WITH IRREVERSIBLE CESSATION OF ALL FUNCTIONS OF THE ENTIRE BRAIN, INCLUDING THE BRAINSTEM, IS DEAD.

The "functions of the entire brain" that are relevant to the diagnosis are those that are clinically ascertainable. Where indicated, the clinical diagnosis is subject to confirmation by laboratory tests as described below. Consultation with a physician experienced in this diagnosis is advisable.

1. *CESSATION* IS RECOGNIZED WHEN EVALUATION DISCLOSES FINDINGS OF a *AND* b:

a. CEREBRAL FUNCTIONS ARE ABSENT, AND...

There must be deep coma, that is, cerebral unreceptivity and unresponsivity. Medical circumstances may require the use of confirmatory studies such as EEG or blood flow study.

b. BRAINSTEM FUNCTIONS ARE ABSENT.

Reliable testing of brainstem reflexes requires a perceptive and experienced physician using adequate stimuli. Pupillary light, corneal, oculocephalic, oculovestibular, oropharyngeal, and respiratory (apnea) reflexes should be tested. When these reflexes cannot be adequately assessed, confirmatory tests are recommended.

Adequate testing for apnea is very important. An accepted method is ventilation with pure oxygen or an oxygen and carbon dioxide mixture for ten minutes before withdrawal of the ventilator, followed by passive flow of oxygen. (This procedure allows PaCO2 to rise without hazardous hypoxia.) Hypercarbia adequately stimulates respiratory effort within thirty seconds when PaCO2 is greater than 60 mmHg. A ten minute period of apnea is usually sufficient to attain this level of hypercarbia. Testing of arterial blood gases can be used to confirm this level. Spontaneous breathing efforts indicate that part of the brainstem is functioning.

Peripheral nervous system activity and spinal cord reflexes may persist after death. True decerebrate or decorticate posturing or seizures are inconsistent with the diagnosis of death.

2. *IRREVERSIBILITY* IS RECOGNIZED WHEN EVALUATION DISCLOSES FINDINGS OF a *AND* b *AND* c:

a. THE CAUSE OF COMA IS ESTABLISHED AND IS SUFFICIENT TO ACCOUNT FOR THE LOSS OF BRAIN FUNCTIONS, AND...

Most difficulties with the determination of death on the basis of neurologic criteria have resulted from inadequate attention to this basic diagnostic prerequisite. In addition to a careful clinical examination and investigation of history, relevant knowledge of causation may be acquired by computed tomographic scan, measurement of core temperature, drug screening, EEG, angiography, or other procedures.

b. THE POSSIBILITY OF RECOVERY OF ANY BRAIN FUNCTIONS IS EXCLUDED, AND...

The most important reversible conditions are sedation, hypothermia, neuromuscular blockade, and shock. In the unusual circumstance where a sufficient cause cannot be established, irreversibility can be reliably inferred only after extensive evaluation for drug intoxication, extended observation, and other testing. A determination that blood flow to the brain is absent can be used to demonstrate a sufficient and irreversible condition.

c. THE CESSATION OF ALL BRAIN FUNCTIONS PERSISTS FOR AN APPROPRIATE PERIOD OF OBSERVATION AND/OR TRIAL OF THERAPY.

Even when coma is known to have started at an earlier time, the absence of all brain functions must be established by an experienced physician at the initiation of the observation period. The duration of observation periods is a matter of clinical judgment, and some physicians recommend shorter or longer periods than those given here.

Except for patients with drug intoxication, hypothermia, young age, or shock, medical centers with substantial experience in diagnosing death neurologically report no cases of brain functions returning following a six hour cessation, documentated by clinical examination and confirmatory EEG. In the absence of confirmatory tests, a period of observation of at least twelve hours is recommended when an irreversible condition is well established. For anoxic brain damage where the extent of damage is more difficult to ascertain, observation for twenty-four hours is generally desirable. In anoxic injury, the observation period may be reduced if a test shows cessation of cerebral blood flow or if an EEG shows electrocerebral silence in an adult patient without drug intoxication, hypothermia, or shock.

Confirmation of clinical findings by EEG is desirable when objective documentation is needed to substantiate the clinical findings. Electrocerebral silence verifies irreversible loss of cortical functions,except in patients with drug intoxiction or hypothermia. (Important technical details are provided in: American Electroencephalographic Society, *Guidelines in EEG 1980*, Section 4: "Minimum Technical Standards for EEG Recording in Suspected Cerebral Death," pp. 19-24, Atlanta, 1980.) When joined with the clinical finding of absent brainstem functions, electrocerebral silence confirms the diagnosis.

Complete cessation of circulation to the normothermic adult brain for more than ten minutes is incompatible with survival of brain tissue. Documentation of this circulatory failure is therefore evidence of death of the entire brain. Four-vessel intracranial angiography is definitive for diagnosing cessation of circulation to the entire brain (both cerebrum and posterior fossa) but entails substantial practical difficulties and risks. Tests are available that assess circulation only in the cerebral hemispheres, namely radioisotope bolus cerebral angiography and gamma camera imaging with radioisotope cerebral angiography. Without complicating conditions, absent cerebral blood flow as measured by these tests, in conjunction with the clinical determination of cessation of all brain functions for at least six hours, is diagnostic of death.

Complicating Conditions

A. Drug and Metabolic Intoxication

Drug intoxication is the most serious problem in the determination of death, especially when multiple drugs are used. Cessation of brain functions caused by the sedative and anesthetic drugs, such as barbiturates, benzodiazepines, meprobamate, methaqualone, and trichloroethylene, may be completely reversible even though they produce clinical cessation of brain functions and electrocerebral silence. In cases where there is any likelihood of sedative presence, toxicology screening for all likely drugs is required. If exogenous intoxication is found, death may not be declared until the intoxicant is metabolized or intracranial circulation is tested and found to have ceased.

Total paralysis may cause unresponsiveness, areflexia, and apnea that closely simulates death. Exposure to drugs such as neuromuscular blocking agents or aminoglycoside antibiotics, and diseases like myasthenia gravis are usually apparent by careful review of the history. Prolonged paralysis after use of succinylcholine chloride and related drugs requires evaluation for pseudo-cholinesterase deficiency. If there is any question, low-dose atropine stimulation, electromyogram, peripheral nerve stimulation, EEG, tests of intracranial circulation, or extended observation, as indicated, will make the diagnosis clear.

In drug-induced coma, EEG activity may return or persist while the patient remains unresponsive, and therefore the EEG may be an important evaluation along with extended observation. If the EEG shows electrocerebral silence, short latency auditory or somatosensory evoked potentials may be used to test brainstem functions, since these potential are unlikely to be affected by drugs.

Some severe illnesses (e.g., hepatic encephalopathy, hyperosmolar coma, and preterminal uremia) can cause deep coma. Before irreversible cessation of brain functions can be determined, metabolic abnormalities should be considered and, if possible, corrected. Confirmatory tests of circulation or EEG may be necessary.

B. Hypothermia

Criteria for reliable recognition of death are not available in the presence of hypothermia (below 32.2°C core temperature). The variables of cerebral circulation in hypothermic patients are not sufficiently well studied to know whether tests of absent or diminished circulation are confirmatory. Hypothermia can mimic brain death by ordinary clinical criteria and can protect against neurologic damage due to hypoxia. Further complications arise since hypothermia also usually precedes and follows death. If these complicating factors make it unclear whether an individual is alive, the only available measure to resolve the issue is to restore normothermia. Hypothermia is not a common cause of difficulty in the determination of death.

C. Children

The brains of infants and young children have increased resistance to damage and may recover substantial functions even after exhibiting unresponsiveness on neurological examination for longer periods than do adults. Physicians should be particularly cautious in applying neurologic criteria to determine death in children younger than five years.

D. Shock

Physicians should also be particularly cautious in applying neurologic criteria to determine death in patients in shock because the reduction in cerebral circulation can render clinical examination and laboratory tests unreliable.

PART FIVE:
Policy Considerations

Section A.
GUIDELINES ON ETHICS COMMITTEES

I. INTRODUCTION

II. GUIDELINES ON IECs

(1) Establishment of an IEC

(2) IEC membership
    (a) Number
    (b) Diversity
    (c) Officers

(3) Schedule

(4) Role of the committee

(5) Confidentiality

(6) Development of the committee

(7) Education
    (a) Committee self-education
    (b) Committee education of others

(8) Policy development

(9) Review of ongoing cases (prospective review)

(10) Insurance coverage

(11) Announcement

PART FIVE:
Policy Considerations

Section A.
GUIDELINES ON ETHICS COMMITTEES

I. INTRODUCTION

At various points the Guidelines recommend the use of an institutional ethics committee (IEC). IECs can perform a number of functions. They can initiate educational programs within the institution. They can also formulate institutional policies and guidelines in ethically sensitive areas, monitor compliance with those policies, and undertake needed policy revision. Finally, they can advise on particular cases and serve as a forum for discussing and resolving disagreement about treatment decisions. In a sense, all of these functions are ways of educating people on specific ethical issues and more generally on the nature and role of medical ethics. An IEC might decide to take on all of these functions, or might decide to take on some but not others.

IECs are actually only one of the mechanisms currently performing these functions. In some institutions an individual ethics consultant or a small team is available for consultation and other functions. Elsewhere, chaplains or other clergy play this role. These Guidelines recommend the use of IECs, but it is more important that some group or person be authorized to fulfill the functions we describe. Education, policy formulation and revision, as well as case review, are necessary institutional elements of ethical decisionmaking, and we strongly encourage all health care institutions to develop some mechanism for performing these functions.

The development of IECs has been characterized by a spirit of experimentation. The Guidelines in this Section are, accordingly, intended to offer suggestions rather than to be rigidly prescriptive. As the President's Commission has noted, society's experience with ethics committees is limited, and we have not yet fully assessed how well they perform their functions. (See BIBLIOGRAPHY.) Yet IECs have engendered widespread enthusiasm and have been established in many places. They are a promising development.

II. GUIDELINES ON IECs

(1) **Establishment of an IEC.** Each hospital, nursing home, hospice, or other health care institution (including home health care agencies) should establish an institutional ethics committee or some other institutional mechanism for providing advice and education on ethical problems. Some institutions may have an ethics consultant, a team of consultants, or clergy who are available for ethics consultations. They may perform many or all of the functions described below, instead of or in coordination with the IEC. Even institutions that have these other resources, however, should consider establishing an IEC, in order to involve a wider spectrum of people in ethics education and the other functions described below. Involving this wider group in case consultations, in particular, may help assure that a broad range of views are considered.

Deciding which body within the institution should formally create and authorize the IEC is a preliminary decision of some significance. Often the choice will be between the institution's board of directors and medical staff. Which is chosen will determine how the IEC is perceived within the institution. It also may affect legal matters, such as the discoverability of IEC records in a legal proceeding, questions that the institution's legal counsel should explore.

An institution starting an ethics committee should commit appropriate resources, including support staff services, supplies, and funds for activities. The institution and third party payers should consider adjustments to reimbursement structures, if necessary, to accommodate this commitment. An institution without the resources to start a full ethics committee should still take action to deal with ethical issues, such as considering a scaled-down version of an ethics committee with just a few people, forming a consortium with other institutions to support a joint ethics committee or ethics consultant, or making sure that at least one person in the institution can advise on ethical issues.

(2) **IEC membership.**

(a) **Number.** The committee should be large enough to represent diverse viewpoints. The IEC may wish to start with a small group of people who are very interested in ethical issues, and then increase the number as the committee matures and gains increasing acceptance in the institution.

(b) **Diversity.** Committee membership should be diverse, including representatives from many areas of the institution and at least one person from outside the institution. Members might include doctors (both senior and junior), nurses, social workers, administrators, lawyers, chaplains or other religious representatives, and people familiar with medical ethics. The institution's legal counsel should not be a member of the committee, but rather should be available to the board of directors, medical staff, or committee for consultation on legal issues. This frees the committee to explore ethical issues without being unduly concerned with legal matters and risk assessment, and provides assurance that IEC recommendations can be reviewed for their legal implications by some other office.

(c) **Officers.** The committee should have a chairperson or co-chairs, plus a vice-chair to assist and to cover when the chair is unavailable.

(3) **Schedule.** In order for the committee to develop competence and become a functioning, known, and trusted body within the institution, meetings should be held regularly and at least monthly.

(4) **Role of the committee.** A new ethics committee should spend some time discussing and clarifying its role. The committee should regard protecting the rights and welfare of patients as its preeminent concern.

(5) **Confidentiality.** The IEC should tackle early the question of which of its proceedings and records will be treated as confidential. There are different views on this. One is that all committee proceedings and records should be treated as confidential, both to protect confidential information about patients and to encourage frank discussion among committee members and institutional staff. Another view is that committee proceedings should be open to wide scrutiny, in part to avoid having a committee rubber-stamp the views of participating health care professionals when it consults on individual cases. The primary consideration in developing a policy should be to protect the confidentiality of patient information. This nonetheless leaves open a variety of possible policies concerning the confidentiality of IEC records and proceedings.

(6) **Development of the committee.** A newly formed committee should educate its members about ethical issues before taking on other tasks. Otherwise, the committee may lack a clear sense of its task, and may not be able to command respect within the institution. The committee also will probably need time to work out its plans and procedures and to develop an atmosphere in which all members feel free to speak their minds.

In keeping with this, a new committee planning to undertake prospective case review (*i.e.,* consultation on individual cases in progress) should initially refrain from that, and instead focus on self-education, policy development, and retrospective review of the ethical issues raised by cases that have already been settled. Indeed, new committees may spend a year or more doing this before they begin any prospective case review.

(7) Education. All IEC functions can be understood as an aspect of education on ethical issues, because they increase awareness of medical ethics. However, there are some methods an IEC can use aimed specifically at educating committee members and others within the institution. These include:

(a) Committee self-education. The IEC may wish to invite speakers to meet with the committee, including members of established committees in other institutions or authorities in the field of ethics. The committee may find it useful to develop a reading list. The committee may also choose to review cases that have been settled so that committee members can discuss the issues without involving or reporting to outsiders. The purpose of this would be to develop facility in identifying ethical issues, and in analyzing and advising on them, and to begin to consider what procedures the IEC may wish to follow if it undertakes the prospective review of ongoing cases. (See Section (9), p. 104.) Another aspect of committee self-education is finding out what ethical issues are arising within the institution. In order to do this, the committee may wish to hold meetings with various groups within the institution.

(b) Committee education of others. The IEC may decide to initiate a variety of efforts within the institution to educate people on specific ethical issues, the nature of medical ethics in general, and the existence and functions of the IEC. The IEC might invite outside speakers on ethics or committee members themselves to address meetings, or the committee might sponsor an event such as Grand Rounds, in-service training, or a day-long symposium.

(8) Policy development. The IEC may be asked to develop institutional policies on ethical issues, or the committee itself may decide that it should develop such policies. Many committees, for instance, have developed policies on "do not resuscitate" orders or on the provision of blood and blood products to Jehovah's Witnesses; some committees have even written broader policies on forgoing life-sustaining treatment. In most or all cases, the IEC will not have the authority to adopt the policy itself, but will be in the position of recommending a policy for adoption by another body within the institution. A committee that undertakes policy development will probably find it worthwhile to communicate with other IECs that have developed policy on the same issue, to collect samples of other policies, and to consult the literature on the topic.

An IEC that develops policy should also consider recommending a system for monitoring compliance with the policy. The committee should play a part in educating people within the institution about the new policy, and periodically consider the need for policy revision.

(9) Review of ongoing cases (prospective review). In order to handle ongoing cases, the IEC will probably find it necessary to develop procedural ground rules and commit them to writing. Those rules should be available to anyone on request, so that people who consider requesting IEC case review can know what process they will be triggering. In addition, patients and surrogates should be informed of the institution's policy on whether IEC review can proceed without consent from the patient or surrogate. The following is a list of some of the issues an IEC should resolve in setting the rules:

(a) Will consulting the ethics committee be optional, or will it be mandatory for certain kinds of cases?

(b) Will the committee's recommendation be advisory, so that following it is optional, or will the committee have decision-making authority?

(c) Who can request that the ethics committee review a problem? Must the patient or surrogate consent to review of the patient's case?

(d) What kind of problems will the committee review? Commonly, an IEC sits to review problems raising significant ethical issues, and refuses problems that are primarily medical or administrative.

(e) Who will determine whether the problem is appropriate for committee review? Will they then call a committee meeting, or will some problems be reviewed by a smaller number of committee members or possibly an individual member? Is there a minimum number of committee members required for a review?

(f) Who will be responsible for collecting the needed information from key individuals? What procedure for discussion will be followed? Will the patient or any other person involved in a case under review be able to meet with members?

(g) Will the reviewing members have to reach a consensus before they render their advice? Who will communicate the recommendation, and to whom? If no consensus can be reached, will that be communicated? Will the committee then identify a range of acceptable approaches or outcomes? Will a note be written in the patient's records stating the outcome of the IEC review?

(h) Will there be regular reports to the full committee of each request for committee review? If a case is reviewed by less than the full committee, will the outcome of the review be reported at the next full committee meeting?

(i) How will the effectiveness and performance of the IEC be evaluated?

(10) **Insurance coverage.** Although lawsuits against IECs will probably be rare, the health care institution should provide insurance coverage for all members of the committee, including members not employed by the facility. Otherwise, concerns about possible legal action against the IEC may unduly influence committee proceedings. The IEC coverage should include attorneys' fees as well as liability, to cover the costs of both defense and judgment.

(11) **Announcement.** A memorandum should be circulated to the staff of the health care institution at least annually, to inform them of the existence of the IEC, its functions, and its availability to consider ethical problems. In addition, we recommend that a brochure be prepared and distributed to all patients and their families or concerned others, conveying the same information.

PART FIVE:
Policy Considerations

Section B.
GUIDELINES ON INSTITUTIONAL POLICIES FOR
PATIENT ADMISSIONS AND TRANSFERS

I. INTRODUCTION

II. GENERAL GUIDELINES ON ADMISSIONS AND TRANSFERS

(1) The need for policies

(2) Admissions

(3) Transfers

III. ADDITIONAL GUIDELINES ON HOSPITALS

(1) Introduction

(2) Admissions to and transfers from hospitals

(3) General in-patient services
   (a) Admissions
   (b) Transfers

(4) Emergency Rooms
   (a) Admissions
   (b) Transfers

(5) Intensive Care Units (ICUs)
   (a) Admissions
   (b) Transfers

IV. ADDITIONAL GUIDELINES ON NURSING HOMES

(1) Introduction

(2) Admissions

(3) Transfers

V. ADDITIONAL GUIDELINES ON HOSPICES

(1) Introduction

(2) Admisssions

(3) Transfers

PART FIVE:
Policy Considerations

Section B.
GUIDELINES ON INSTITUTIONAL POLICIES FOR
PATIENT ADMISSIONS AND TRANSFERS

I. INTRODUCTION

Whether a patient receives or forgoes a life-sustaining treatment depends to some extent on the health care setting. The distinctive character of different health care settings affects the kinds of treatment offered. A decision to admit a patient to a particular health care setting is also a decision about the level of medical care that will be available.

Ideally, there should not be a rigid correlation between the patient's setting and the kind of care available; a patient should have a variety of treatment options, including the option to forgo treatments, without having to change settings. There currently is, however, a correlation between setting and available care. In a hospital—particularly an acute care hospital—certain kinds of life-sustaining treatment may be routinely provided. In a long-term care facility certain life-sustaining treatments may rarely be provided. In order to plan for treatment, patients and health care professionals need to know about institutional policies on admissions and transfers, on the kinds of treatment available, and on forgoing life-sustaining treatment. These Guidelines present a general ethical framework to assist hospitals, nursing homes, and hospices in developing such policies; the Guidelines do not offer specific policies for adoption.

Patients need to develop more control over where they receive care. Since the patient's setting affects the kind of health care offered, it is important to seek the patient's agreement for admission and transfer* whenever possible. However, it would be impossible as a practical matter to require consent to transfer as we require consent to treatment—that would mean that patients could stay in health care institutions until they chose to leave. Our health care system would probably not be able to function.

---

*Throughout this Section the term "transfer" applies to moving the patient from one setting to another, whether the new setting is within the same health care institution, in another institution, or at home. A variety of words are used to refer to such placement. Because these Guidelines most often apply to gravely ill patients, and most of these patients will literally be "transferred" to the care of other health care professionals or another institution, we use that term.

It is also important to ensure continuity of care when a patient transfers from one setting to another. Otherwise treatment decisions already made may not be communicated, and the process of developing a plan of treatment may be disrupted. (See PART THREE.) We make several recommendations to promote continuity of care.

II. GENERAL GUIDELINES ON ADMISSIONS AND TRANSFERS

(1) **The need for policies.** Health care institutions should develop written policies on admission and transfer, and communicate these to patients and surrogates, preferably before admission, to permit planning to the extent possible for the setting of the patient's care. Institutions should also develop written policies concerning any restrictions they place on using or forgoing life-sustaining treatments, and should make these publicly available. In this way patients and surrogates will be informed about what entering the setting entails for the patient's medical treatment. Policies should ensure, as much as possible, that patients and surrogates can decide among treatment options and forgo specific treatments without the patient having to be transferred to a different setting. Policies should also be flexible and open to revision in light of improved therapeutic interventions, the needs of patients, and institutional concerns.

In both admission and transfer, the primary concern should be the patient's welfare. Institutions should attempt to eliminate contrary incentives. They should inform patients and surrogates of those incentives that persist.

(2) **Admissions.** Generally, patients who should be admitted to a health care institution, or to a setting within one, are those who require the services offered there and who cannot be better cared for in another setting.

Whenever possible, before admission or soon after, health care professionals should ascertain the patient's preferences concerning kinds and degrees of care. Admission to a health care institution or a setting within one generally should not be conditioned on a patient's or surrogate's acceptance of a particular life-sustaining treatment. Similarly, the fact that a patient has an advance directive, or that the patient or surrogate has decided to forgo a life-sustaining treatment, ordinarily should not prevent the patient's admission to a health care institution or any setting within the institution or cause transfer out of one. When patients have an advance directive or a written treatment plan (see PART THREE), these should be entered into the medical records and should be readily accessible, so that health care professionals can implement them.

(3) **Transfers.** A patient should be transferred to another institution, or to another setting within an institution, or to his or her own home, when the following criteria are met: more appropriate care is available there, the benefits of the transfer outweigh the risks to the patient, the receiving setting or institution accepts the patient, and the patient or surrogate is informed of the reasons for the proposed transfer.

Before the transfer, the patient or surrogate should receive an explanation of the need for the transfer, any risks it entails, and the alternatives to transfer. The patient or surrogate should be informed of protections afforded to the patient under the pertinent rules, policy, and law. The patient or surrogate should be invited to respond to the transfer proposal; if he or she objects after discussing the matter, appropriate review should be made available. Review might involve referral to an institutional ethics committee or other institutional mechanism for advising on ethical issues.

Whenever a patient is transferred, health care providers should, if possible, enable the patient to retain the same responsible health care professional. In any case, the responsible professional should prepare a transfer summary and convey it to the health care professionals in the new setting. The document should include any information needed for continuity, and at a minimum should: state the reason for transfer; summarize decisions already made to receive or forgo treatment, particularly life-sustaining treatment; indicate what treatment plan, if any, has been developed; and note the existence of any advance directives and the identity of the patient's surrogate.

III. ADDITIONAL GUIDELINES ON HOSPITALS

(1) **Introduction.** Hospitals emphasize acute care, often involving sophisticated medical technology. Even though hospitals have other goals and services, such as diagnosis, rehabilitation, and amelioration of the effects of disease, the "rescue" atmosphere is pervasive—in other words, the impetus is great to use any treatment that will fend off death. This is reinforced by current reimbursement policies, which provide financial incentives to place patients in diagnostic categories that call for the greatest degree of acute care possible. Many patients welcome this "rescue" ethos. However, patients who wish to forgo some forms of life-sustaining treatment may find it less desirable.

(2) **Admissions to and transfers from hospitals.** When a patient is admitted to a hospital, that admission is to a particular service or unit of the institution; transfer from the hospital is similarly from a particular service or unit. Nevertheless, the institution as a whole has a responsibility for the care of patients who are admitted. To discharge this responsibility, hospitals should make certain that one health care professional is assigned primary responsibility for each patient who is admitted. That professional should ensure that continuity of care is provided.

(3) **General in-patient services.**

(a) **Admissions.** Patients who will benefit from the diagnosis and treatment of illnesses or conditions that have the potential for cure, arrest, remission, or palliation using medical or surgical treatment are candidates for admission to the general in-patient services of a hospital.

The following persons should generally not be admitted to hospitals because they can better be cared for in other health care settings. They should be offered referrals to these other settings and assistance in arranging care.

1. Non-hospitalized persons who, while capable of making decisions, have indicated that they do not wish to be admitted to a hospital to receive life-sustaining measures, or whose surrogates so indicate on their behalf.

2. Persons who require nursing care at home or in a long-term care facility, when those options are available and more appropriate.

(b) **Transfers.** When a patient is transferred from one service to another or to a separate unit within the hospital, a written transfer summary need not be prepared. However, the responsible health care professional should make sure that all relevant information is conveyed to the admitting service or unit, including all of the information that would be included in a transfer summary. (See Section II (3), p. 110.)

(4) **Emergency Rooms.**

(a) **Admissions.** All patients who present themselves or are brought to Emergency Rooms with conditions that are life-threatening should be examined and evaluated by a health care professional. Some of these patients will require admission to the hospital through the Emergency Room. The criteria for admission to the relevant service or unit of the hospital should apply. However, patients should not be refused admission to the hospital through the Emergency Room unless they can get appropriate care elsewhere and their condition has stabilized.

The source of payment should not govern whether patients are admitted to Emergency Rooms. Economic considerations should not be allowed to deprive patients of needed care. Regional arrangements should be made for the ongoing treatment of patients admitted to Emergency Rooms, so that those who are unable to pay have access to needed care.

(b) Transfers. Before patients are transferred, they should receive all immediately necessary care, their condition should be stabilized as defined by professional standards (except when they are transferred within the institution), and precautions should be taken so that the move does not harm them.

(5) Intensive Care Units (ICUs).

(a) Admissions. The following patients are candidates for admission to ICUs when it is consistent with their treatment preferences and goals: critically ill patients who require life support for organ system failure that may be reversible or remediable; patients with irreversible organ system failure who cannot be treated appropriately in another setting; patients at risk of developing life-threatening complications who require monitoring or treatment; and patients who are receiving a trial period of monitoring and treatment when there is doubt about the prognosis or the effectiveness of therapy. A decision to forgo a life-sustaining treatment (such as cardiopulmonary resuscitation) should not preclude other forms of treatment and admission to the ICU. Admission should be subject to constraints imposed by the availability of space, equipment, and personnel, the needs of patients already in the unit, and the needs of others who are also candidates for admission.

Patients who generally should not be admitted to ICUs include:

1. Patients with documented irreversible cessation of all functions of the entire brain, except those whose cardiopulmonary functions are being maintained for the purpose of organ donation or for other reasons as set forth in PART FOUR: Section (3), p. 89.

2. Patients who have been firmly diagnosed as irreversibly unconscious.

3. Patients with irreversible illness who are near death, except in unusual circumstances when intensive care may provide a form of palliation or pain relief.

4. Patients who, while capable of making decisions, have requested that they not receive intensive care or its equivalent; patients whose advance directives or treatment plans indicate that they would not desire intensive care in their present circumstances; and patients whose surrogates refuse intensive care for them.

Admission to ICUs should be based on established medical criteria that are grounded in accepted principles of triage based on the severity of illness and predictors of outcome and morbidity (the APACHE system is one example of a critical care guide—see BIBLIOGRAPHY). These criteria should be subject to continuous reevaluation in light of improved therapeutic interventions and prognostic indicators.

Patients are entitled to refuse admission to an ICU, even when doing so puts them at risk of death. Patients should not, however, be able to require admission to an ICU. A request by a patient or surrogate for admission to an ICU may be denied if admission would be medically inappropriate for the patient, detrimental to patients already in the unit, or contrary to the admission criteria. Should a patient be denied admission to an ICU, the patient or surrogate should receive an explanation of the reasons for the denial. They should also be informed of protections afforded to the patient under the pertinent rules, policy, and law. Appropriate review should be made available to patients or surrogates who object to this decision. Review might involve referral to an institutional ethics committee or other institutional mechanism for advising on ethical issues.

(b) **Transfers.** Patients should be transferred from ICUs to another setting within the hospital or another institution when intensive care will no longer benefit them, either because they have improved to a point where intensive care is no longer necessary or because they have deteriorated to a point where it no longer offers reasonable promise of benefit. Sometimes it is necessary to transfer one patient out of the ICU to make room for another patient. Such triage is ethically appropriate when the criteria are written and generally accepted.

Patients who are eligible for transfer from ICUs may remain when there is room and:

1. they will die immediately, and it is preferable that they die in the familiar surroundings of the ICU; or

2. they will die in the near future, and they and their surrogate, family, and concerned friends need a short period of time to adjust to this; or

3. they will die in the near future, and their comfort requires the management of some technology most skillfully handled in the ICU.

IV. ADDITIONAL GUIDELINES ON NURSING HOMES

(1) **Introduction.** Nursing homes are places of residence for those with physical and mental disabilities who require assistance in the daily course of living. These facilities usually do not have extensive capacities to detect and treat life-threatening conditions. Three groups of patients tend to enter nursing homes. One group enters from the hospital with short-term problems, and leaves within a few months. Patients in this group usually wish to have life-sustaining treatment administered to them should they have an unexpected medical crisis, and may require transfer back to the hospital in such an event. Another group enters for short-term care prior to death. Such patients generally do not wish to have life-sustaining treatment administered. The third group consists of long-term nursing home residents who have no immediate family member able to care for them at home, or for whom continued home care is no longer a viable option. Entry into a nursing home can mean a substantial loss of personal autonomy for these persons. They are leaving a familiar living environment to enter a new and strange one. They usually have little choice in selecting their health care professionals, and those professionals may not be familiar with them and their preferences. There is a pressing need to ascertain the treatment wishes of individuals in this group.

(2) **Admissions.** Those who require skilled nursing care or a protected environment and assistance with daily activities are candidates for admission to nursing homes. Medicare and state Medicaid programs set criteria for admitting covered individuals. The trend has been toward limiting admissions to individuals who are severely incapacitated. This greatly restricts long-term care options for those who are moderately incapacitated. There is a need to develop options for these individuals.

Patients who generally should not be admitted to nursing homes include:

(a) those who currently need and wish to receive life-sustaining treatment that cannot be provided in the nursing home;

(b) those who can live at home with in-home services actually available to them, without incurring unreasonable risk or burden; and

(c) those who need a type of care that the particular nursing home cannot provide.

In addition, some people cannot be cared for in a nursing home without endangering themselves or others, and so should not be admitted. Such a determination depends on the characteristics of the particular patient and the nursing home in question.

Because nursing homes are long-term residential institutions, patients who have not developed advance directives before admission should be encouraged to do so. Patients should be asked in particular under what circumstances they would desire transfer to a hospital, because of the common use of life-sustaining treatments in that setting. When the nursing home develops a treatment plan for each patient, the patient should participate in this process. (See PART THREE.)

(3) Transfers.

Transfers within nursing homes. For seriously or terminally ill individuals, unnecessary intra-institutional transfer may lead to additional disorientation and confusion, worsening pain and suffering. Such transfers should be avoided, and regulatory and reimbursement policies for skilled and intermediate care should support non-transfer in such situations.

Transfers from nursing homes. When a patient is being transferred from a nursing home, the nursing home and patient or surrogate should reach an agreement about the conditions under which the patient will return to the nursing home.

To hospitals. Hospitalization should be recommended when consistent with the patient's preferences and values and when medically indicated, such as in an emergency, when needed to treat or diagnose the patient, when recommended for the patient's health, or when the comfort of other nursing home patients requires it. Should hospitalization be contemplated in order to provide a painful or invasive intervention for a patient whose illness is following an irreversible course toward death, and should the hospitalization seem likely to result in the patient's severe disorientation, transfer should be recommended only when the clinical benefits will outweigh these special risks and the other risks of treatment.

To hospices. People expected to die within the time period specified by hospice admission rules may be transferred to a hospice unit within the nursing home, a hospice in a separate institution, or a hospice that cares for people in their homes, for the purpose of relieving their symptoms and pain and suffering. Some nursing homes provide a hospice style of care so that no transfer within or outside the institution is necessary.

To home. Individuals who no longer need skilled nursing care and who can live at home with some supportive assistance without unreasonable risk, may be transferred from nursing homes to their own homes or other living situations, when appropriate home health care services can be provided.

V. ADDITIONAL GUIDELINES ON HOSPICES

(1) **Introduction.** A decision to enter a hospice program is ordinarily a decision to forgo life-sustaining treatment and to allow death to come in a supportive setting that focuses on symptom control. Hospice care provides not only attention to the physical pain and suffering of a dying person, but also to emotional and spiritual pain and suffering. Patients who enter hospice programs do not receive vigorous curative interventions, but they do receive palliative care and pain relief designed to make their remaining life more comfortable. Hospices may provide services at the homes of individuals, in separate institutions, within hospitals, or within nursing homes.

The rules currently governing Medicare reimbursement for hospice care may make it difficult for hospice patients to obtain life-sustaining treatment in acute care facilities if it becomes warranted. Those rules may discourage hospices from placing patients in costly acute care settings or accepting very ill patients. Unless these rules are changed, hospices should inform potential patients or their surrogates about the rules and conscientiously review treatment decisions to which patients or surrogates object.

(2) **Admissions.** Individuals with a diagnosis of terminal illness and an estimated life expectancy that meets hospice admission criteria (usually six months or less) are eligible for hospice care. Life expectancy is notoriously difficult to estimate; in estimating life span some degree of flexibility is necessary to afford dying patients access to the palliative care and pain relief that hospices offer. The consent of the patient and usually of a person who will help to care for the patient is also necessary for admission.

Some hospices will accept only patients who have exhausted all curative treatment. This admission requirement could unreasonably force curative attempts on patients who wish to decline them.

(3) Transfers. When a patient is being transferred from a hospice, the hospice and patient or surrogate should reach an agreement about the conditions under which the patient will return to the hospice. A patient ordinarily should only be transferred out of a hospice in an unexpected situation and to receive treatment for a specific problem (for example, if a patient requires hospitalization to treat a broken bone).

PART FIVE:
Policy Considerations

Section C.
THE USE OF ECONOMIC CONSIDERATIONS IN
DECISIONS CONCERNING LIFE-SUSTAINING
TREATMENTS

I. INTRODUCTION

II. ASSESSING THE VALUE OF TREATMENT: COSTWORTHY CARE

III. THE ROLE OF HEALTH CARE PROFESSIONALS IN PROVIDING COSTWORTHY CARE

IV. WAYS TO DEVELOP POLICIES

V. GUIDELINES ON DEVELOPING A COSTWORTHY APPROACH TO INDIVIDUAL TREATMENT DECISIONS

(1) Reasons to develop a costworthy approach

(2) Patients' assessments of whether treatment options are costworthy
  (a) When making treatment choices
  (b) When purchasing health insurance
  (c) When developing advance directives

(3) Avoiding inequitable allocation in individual patient care

(4) Limiting available treatment options as a matter of policy

PART FIVE:
Policy Considerations

Section C.
THE USE OF ECONOMIC CONSIDERATIONS IN
DECISIONS CONCERNING LIFE-SUSTAINING
TREATMENTS

I. INTRODUCTION

There is currently no policy available on national, local, or institutional levels that would ethically justify the use of economic considerations in decisions concerning life-sustaining treatment. This is partly because the debate about the ethical role of economic considerations is not nearly as well developed as the debate about many other issues considered in these Guidelines. There is no consensus about the just use of economic considerations in health care in general that can be formulated here, and then applied to life-sustaining treatments in particular. This Section of the Guidelines, therefore, is meant to advance the debate on ethical uses of economic considerations, with special reference to decisions about life-sustaining treatment. For the most part, it does not offer specific guidelines for health care professionals and institutions, but instead provides both a general ethical framework within which policies could be developed, and procedural recommendations for devising such policies.

The inclusion of a Section on economic considerations in Guidelines on forgoing treatment is not meant to suggest that it is necessary or appropriate to reduce care for patients who are dying or forgoing life-sustaining treatment. Some people argue that patients at the end of their lives now receive excessive and overly expensive care, but the data do not support this. Those near death probably do receive a higher proportion of expensive medical care than others. However, available studies do not indicate that this care is generally inappropriate, wasteful, or unjust. Therefore, there is at present no justification for embarking on a stringent program to ration life-sustaining medical care for those who are near the end of life in order to contain costs.

At the same time, individual patients may wish to take into account the costs of various kinds of medical treatment when they make treatment choices, arrange for health care insurance, and prepare advance directives. (See PART THREE.) Methods should be devised to enable such patients to do so. Patients should be given the opportunity to state their views about those circumstances in which they would consider intensive care and other life-sustaining treatment to be worth the cost, and those circumstances in which they would not.

On governmental and institutional levels coordinated policies should be developed to identify not only wasteful, useless, and harmful treatment, but also those forms of treatment whose benefits do not justify large financial outlays, in light of the alternative possible uses of those resources. Policies must be designed so that the goal being served is legitimate and the means used are likely to accomplish that goal. A wide range of reasonable and just choices are possible. Fair procedures should be used in developing policies, due consideration given to relevant information and interests, and institutional policies should be subject to accountability.

The health care professional caring for an individual patient should *not* be involved in cutting costs or rationing scarce resources at the bedside for the benefit of society, unless it is in accordance with institutional or governmental policy. No such policy now exists. To engage in hidden rationing would risk arbitrary and unfair decisions, not because caregivers would necessarily choose inappropriately, but because such decisions would not be based on principled and explicit policies. If explicit and ethical policies are developed by means of procedures that are open, informed, and fair, health care providers might be justified in limiting their treatments to patients in accordance with such policies. This would be in keeping with the long-standing concern of the health care professions with issues of justice and societal well-being, as well as with patient autonomy and well-being.

In striving to contain medical care costs, it is important to avoid discriminating against the critically ill and dying, to shun invidious comparisons of the economic value of various individuals to society, and to refuse to abandon patients and hasten death to save money. Policies must not worsen the already substantial inequities in access to health care. Many people in this country—including the poor, unemployed, and aged—do not have access to adequate care. There is a pressing need to solve this problem; cutting costs and allocating care should not exacerbate it. Some cost-containment strategies may already be depriving some patients of care that should be available. It is critical to remember that cutting costs is only part of the problem—making sure that individuals are not wrongly deprived of care is equally important.

II. ASSESSING THE VALUE OF TREATMENT: COSTWORTHY CARE

Policies should be developed on governmental and institutional levels to identify those forms of treatment that are costworthy. It is necessary, that is, to begin to identify as a matter of public policy those forms of health care whose benefits are worth their costs in comparison with alternative uses of the same resources. The concept of costworthy care, as used in these Guidelines, does not measure the benefits of treatment in terms of human capital or productivity, nor does it view the number of life-years or quality-adjusted years saved as the ultimate criterion. Instead, the concept of costworthy care assesses the value of medical treatments for patients in terms of the sacrifice that such treatments entail by requiring us to give up other forms of health care, or other legitimate individual and societal goods.

At the individual level, patients should be asked to begin identifying treatment that is costworthy to them, by assessing whether the benefits of various treatments are worth their costs when compared with other uses that they might make of the same resources. Most patients pay only part of the costs of their care at the time of utilization because they have some form of insurance; questions about the costworthiness of expenses borne by third-party payers should be handled at an institutional and governmental level. However, the out-of-pocket costs to individuals can still be significant. Patients, whether insured or not, are legitimately concerned about the financial expense to them of various life-sustaining treatment options. A growing number of reports describe the immense costs of this treatment to some patients in their last days of life and the plight of families forced into financial straits. In some instances, it is questionable whether the patients would have wanted this treatment had they been apprised at an opportune time about the expense and the small probability of benefit. Patients may decide that certain treatments—even those that are life-sustaining—are not sufficiently promising or beneficial to warrant their costs. Patients may reject even treatments with a substantial probability of medical benefit.

Patients' decisions about the costworthiness of care may be unjustly skewed, however, for those who are uninsured or unable to pay. As a matter of public policy, this group should be provided with a decent and adequate level of care without undue cost to them. Only then will the most vulnerable members of society be in a position to evaluate whether their care is costworthy.

Different persons reasonably disagree over the weight and importance they assign to particular treatment outcomes and in their assessments of costworthiness. On the level of individual decisions by patients, it is important to tolerate this diversity of views as part of respect for patient autonomy. However, on the level of social policy it is important to strive for some societal consensus. Currently there is no generally recognized way to apply the concept of costworthiness. There is no agreed upon measure of costs in comparison to benefits and the value of alternative uses of the resources. It is also difficult to determine what alternative uses would be made of resources conserved by cutting the costs of medical care. The Guidelines can nevertheless offer some suggestions on what sort of treatment is costworthy and can recommend basic procedures to follow in order to identify such treatment and begin to formulate policy.

Treatment that is wasteful, useless, or harmful is not costworthy. If a treatment does not benefit individual patients or promote social well-being, then it cannot be worth its costs. Some forms of treatment may benefit patients, but perhaps not sufficiently to be considered costworthy. These have been referred to as "marginally beneficial" treatments, and there are many kinds. Some offer significant benefit to very few patients at substantial cost; some offer slight benefit to large numbers of patients at substantial cost; and there are other variations.

An ethic that aims to provide costworthy care cannot assume that any medical intervention that offers some benefit, no matter how marginal, should be provided regardless of its cost to others. Nor can it, at the other extreme, advocate adopting any plan of allocation that maximizes net benefits to the greatest number of patients at the least cost, regardless of how individual patient benefits are distributed. Instead, such an ethic must ask whether treatment that is marginally beneficial is costworthy in light of some satisfactory balance between benefit to the individual patient and alternative uses of these resources. This is not solely an economic policy question. Medical issues such as the efficacy and necessity of treatment, and moral issues such as the requirements of justice, must enter into this determination.

Adopting such a policy would not necessarily mean eliminating all forms of expensive life-sustaining treatment. This society places a high value on human beings and their lives. Undoubtedly, many forms of life-sustaining treatment would be seen as well worth their costs in comparison with other forms of health care or other goods that could be provided in their stead. Patients who would be denied marginally beneficial life-sustaining treatments as a result of such policies, however, should receive some assurance that the savings achieved will be used to benefit others in ways that are just and equitable. Current strategies to constrain the rising costs of health care provide no such assurance.

III. THE ROLE OF HEALTH CARE PROFESSIONALS IN PROVIDING COSTWORTHY CARE

Health care professionals have an obligation to act for the good of their patients. Many have tended to regard the cost of treatment to the patient as irrelevant to this obligation. In recent decades, with various forms of health care insurance and third party payments widely available, health care professionals did not usually have to consider the financial welfare of their patients. Today, however, the situation is changing as government, private insurers, and employers are setting limits on health care coverage. The increasing use of co-payments and deductibles is shifting more out-of-pocket costs onto patients. Health care professionals are being asked now to consider the costs of the treatment that they recommend to patients in light of the patients' financial well-being, and to help patients assess whether the treatment is costworthy.

Many health care professionals find it distasteful to discuss the costs of care with patients, especially the cost of life-sustaining treatment. But such discussions are not at odds with the traditions of the health care professions. Before private insurance, Medicare, and Medicaid, health care professionals felt obligated to ascertain whether certain treatments were too expensive for their patients in view of the proportion of benefits to burdens. They did not believe that they were professionally obligated to provide all treatments that yielded some benefit, no matter how marginal, regardless of cost. Health care professionals ought to discuss whether care is costworthy with patients who are concerned about it, and to provide information about alternative treatments. They also have a professional duty to resist reimbursement incentives (including those created by the advent of prospective payment) and other inducements to ration medical care in their own financial interests, rather than in the interests of their patients.

Many believe that a patient-centered ethic requires health care professionals to disregard the effect of one patient's treatment on the welfare of other patients. To some extent this is the case; the health care professional should not engage in cost-cutting or rationing at the bedside unless the patient requests it or explicit institutional or governmental policy requires it. But if future policies require professionals to provide only that care which society considers costworthy, they may have to refrain from providing some treatments and tests that might benefit the immediate patient for the good of other patients with whom they have no connection.

Costworthy policies for delivering health care could well limit professionals' discretion. They would still exercise their professional judgment, but they alone would not determine which treatment options would be available. Administrators would have some control over treatment allocation and would set limits to clinical options and the decisions of individual professionals. Professional discretion is currently limited by cost-containment strategies; treatment limitations based on costworthy policies would add ethical considerations related to justice and equity.

IV. WAYS TO DEVELOP POLICIES

In developing policies on costworthy care at the institutional and governmental levels, there is a danger that those without the means to pay for health care will be forced to carry the burden of cost containment. Those who are uninsured or at risk of bankruptcy because of their medical care costs should not be barred from receiving medical treatment. Indeed, those without the means to pay should be assured of a decent and adequate level of health care as a matter of public policy. Further public discussion is needed to develop an acceptable definition of adequate health care.

To develop policies on costworthy care, it is important to develop adequate data and predictors. Without knowing whether patients are being helped or harmed by various forms of treatment, in what numbers, to what extent, and at what cost, costworthy treatment cannot be identified. The distribution of benefits and burdens among different categories of patients is also significant information to gather. There is a pressing need to determine whether proposed treatments and those currently in use will change the outcome of medical care, and to obtain information about their real costs in order to evaluate whether they are costworthy.

As that information is collected, health care institutions of all kinds — as well as public bodies — have a responsibility to begin discussing whether various forms of treatment are costworthy, as a step toward the development of coordinated institutional and public policy. It is important to explore the benefits of a certain health care expenditure relative to the benefits that would result from expending an equivalent amount of public resources in another area of health care, or on a potentially competing social welfare item (for example, education), or in another area altogether (for example, foreign aid or defense). Identifying harmful, useless, and wasteful treatments should be the first consideration. Then marginally beneficial treatments that are not costworthy should be identified. Criteria that should *not* be used for limiting treatment and allocating health care resources should also be identified.

To pursue these discussions, public bodies at state and national levels could utilize administrative agencies already in place or specially appointed committees composed of health care professionals, regulators, financers, and patients, among others, to begin developing some reasoned, broad, and just consensus on costworthy care. Within institutions a committee could be appointed for this purpose whose members are especially knowledgeable about the medical, economic, and ethical issues. The members of such a committee should include but not be limited to physicians, nurses, administrators, and patients.

V. GUIDELINES ON DEVELOPING A COSTWORTHY APPROACH TO INDIVIDUAL TREATMENT DECISIONS

(1) **Reasons to develop a costworthy approach.** A patient-oriented and costworthy approach to decisions about medical treatment avoids imposing great financial burdens on patients without their consent. It can enhance patients' autonomy by allowing them to determine whether the benefits of treatment are worth their costs to the patient in view of alternative uses of resources. It can enhance patients' well-being by giving them the opportunity to reject forms of treatment that they consider too expensive.

(2) **Patients' assessments of whether treatment options are costworthy.** When they wish and when feasible, patients should have the opportunity to evaluate which forms of health care available to them are costworthy. They may wish to address this question in at least three major circumstances:

(a) **When making treatment choices.** In deciding whether to receive or forgo various forms of treatment, including life-sustaining treatment, patients may wish to consider what financial burdens the treatment will impose on them and others. Health care professionals should inform patients of the costs of various options, if they wish to consider this.

(b) **When purchasing health care insurance.** When patients investigate the options available in health insurance packages, they should be informed of the kind, extent, and costs of coverage.

(c) **When developing advance directives.** If individuals develop advance directives (see PART THREE), they may wish to take into account whether various forms of treatment are costworthy from their perspective and instruct health care professionals accordingly.

(3) Avoiding inequitable allocation in individual patient care. In caring for an individual patient, a health care professional should not cut costs or ration scarce medical resources, except in accordance with the patient's wishes or explicit policy at the institutional or governmental level.

(4) Limiting available treatment options as a matter of policy. In some instances, individuals may desire a treatment that has been evaluated as not costworthy as a matter of public or institutional policy. When such policies have been developed according to procedures and standards that are reasonable and just by government or by institutions, it is ethically justifiable for health care professionals to follow such policies and to refuse to provide this treatment. Patients should be informed of the policy before entering the health care institution and told of alternative settings in which they might receive such treatment.

PART SIX:
Special Problems

**I. TERMINATING TREATMENT, ACTIVE
VOLUNTARY EUTHANASIA, AND
ASSISTING SUICIDE**

**II. WITHHOLDING AND WITHDRAWING
TREATMENT**

**III. DECISIONMAKING CAPACITY AND
COMPETENCE**

IV. "QUALITY OF LIFE"

V. AGE AS A FACTOR IN DECISIONMAKING

**VI. ACCOMMODATING RELIGIOUS VALUES
AND BELIEFS**

PART SIX:
Special Problems

This final Part elaborates on six key issues. There are any number of issues raised by the termination of treatment that could be discussed. These six have been chosen because they are important subjects of ongoing debate.

I. TERMINATING TREATMENT, ACTIVE VOLUNTARY EUTHANASIA, AND ASSISTING SUICIDE

These Guidelines firmly endorse the right of a patient with decisionmaking capacity, or a surrogate for a patient who lacks capacity, to decide to forgo any life-sustaining medical treatment. That right is grounded in the importance of respecting a patient's self-determination, particularly on a question as significant as the manner and time of death. Whether treatment and continued life is on balance a benefit to the patient will depend on the nature of the life that can be offered and the patient's particular goals and values. The patient, or surrogate acting for the patient, should apply those goals and values in making this determination.

Some persons who accept this right of patients to decide to forgo treatment are concerned nevertheless that the values supporting it, and in particular self-determination, necessarily imply that voluntary euthanasia and assisted suicide are also justified. We disagree. Medical tradition and customary practice distinguish in a broadly acceptable fashion between the refusal of medical interventions and intentionally causing death or assisting suicide.

This tradition does not hold the health care professional morally responsible for the death of a patient when life-sustaining treatment is refused and the professional's purpose is not to cause death, but to honor the refusal. Similarly, the tradition defends the administration of a treatment that may hasten death when the professional's purpose is to relieve pain and suffering and the patient or surrogate consents. By contrast, this tradition does not permit administering massive doses of sedatives for the purpose of bringing about death, even if requested by the patient or surrogate.

Such distinctions may raise complex and controversial issues in some cases. Whatever the intrinsic moral differences may or may not be, however, there are substantial policy reasons that support distinguishing between the refusal of treatment and active euthanasia or "mercy killing" or assisted suicide. The authority of health care professionals to help patients decide about life-sustaining treatment, and then to carry out those decisions, is an awesome power. Society is quite reasonably interested in making sure that the power is carefully limited and used wisely and responsibly. There are widespread public concerns about vesting such power over life and death with any group, including health care professionals. There are also concerns about how that power might be misused or misapplied to cases, even when the intentions are good. In order to respond to these concerns, it is a reasonable policy to draw a line between a patient's right to decide about medical treatment, on one side, and euthanasia or "mercy killing" and assisted suicide, on the other.

When patients or surrogates refuse treatment, criminal prosecution of health care professionals for acceding to those treatment decisions is extremely rare. Most people, including prosecutors, judges, and jurors, consider motivation in their assessments. Ordinarily, when a patient chooses to forgo treatment there is no element of willful self-destruction, only the recognition that a further medical treatment would be unduly burdensome; when the health care professional complies with the patient's or surrogate's choice, the intent is to respect and support, not destroy the patient. Forgoing treatment also is commonly less certain to result in death than the behavior at issue in ordinary prosecuted cases, such as shooting or stabbing. Furthermore, even when a medical intervention hastens death, the means used are those ordinarily used in treatment—analgesics, sedatives, or anesthetics— not those associated with criminals—poisons, guns, or knives.

If the traditional line between patients or their surrogates making treatment choices and euthanasia or "mercy killing" or assisted suicide limits the self-determination of some patients, that may be worthwhile in order to assure that other patients' rights to forgo treatment are not abused and appropriate limits are maintained. Some argue that it would be more humane in some instances to carry out active euthanasia or "mercy killing" or to assist suicide rather than to allow patients to die slowly in pain and suffering. This argument, based on mercy and concern about the prolongation of suffering, should not be minimized. Yet its proponents overlook the potential of contemporary medicine to provide palliation and pain relief to those who are dying. If medicine's capacity for relieving pain and suffering were fully tapped, there would probably be no significant foundation for this argument. Health care professionals have a moral duty to provide adequate palliative care and pain relief, even if such care shortens the patient's life.

II. WITHHOLDING AND WITHDRAWING TREATMENT

Health care professionals often find it more acceptable not to start treatment than to stop a treatment already under way. The psychological distinction between not starting and stopping is widely recognized. Yet it is also widely acknowledged that both not starting treatment and stopping it—withholding and withdrawing—can be morally acceptable. The difference between them is not one of moral importance.

When a patient or surrogate decides that a proposed treatment and the life it offers will impose undue burdens, the patient or the surrogate should be entitled to refuse the treatment, based on the patient's right to self-determination. Health care professionals act in a morally appropriate way in respecting that choice and not starting treatment. Similarly, when a patient or surrogate in collaboration with the responsible health care professional decides that a treatment under way and the life it provides have become more burdensome than beneficial to the patient, that is sufficient reason to stop. There is no ethical requirement that once treatment has been initiated, it must continue against the patient's wishes or when the surrogate determines that it is more burdensome than beneficial from the patient's perspective. In fact, imposing treatment in such circumstances violates the patient's right to self-determination.

There is actually a strong reason to prefer stopping treatment over not starting it in some cases. Often there is uncertainty about the efficacy of a proposed treatment, or the burdens and benefits it will impose on the patient. It is preferable then to start the treatment and later stop if it is ineffective or overly burdensome from the patient's perspective—to use time-limited trials as we recommend in PART ONE: Section (6) (a), p. 30—rather than not to start the treatment for fear that stopping will be impossible or unethical. Not starting in these circumstances could deprive the patient of beneficial treatment that the patient might find desirable.

Some health care professionals worry that stopping treatment, even when ethically justifiable, may constitute wrongful killing. Stopping seems more obvious than not starting treatment, and so prompts more fear of legal consequences; to begin a rescue, and then to stop while a patient's death ensues, would seem to entail moral responsiblity for that death. Certainly it would be wrong to stand by and needlessly allow a patient's death, but this is not the case here. Instead, treatment is withdrawn because it is unwanted. When health care professionals stop treating patients for good moral reasons, and those patients subsequently die, the professionals are not morally culpable. They end treatment in good faith, just as they began it. In so doing, health care professionals acknowledge that unwanted treatment should not be imposed on patients.

Some health care professionals may find it difficult to stop life-sustaining treatment because they have been trained to do everything possible to support life. Stopping such treatment seems to them a professional wrong. Yet ending that treatment for good reason does not violate the obligations of health care professionals. To the contrary, it acknowledges that in some cases medical treatment is no longer regarded as beneficial by the patient, and that health care professionals then have a duty to consider how best to end the treatment. When treatment is unwanted, stopping acknowledges that patients, or their surrogates acting for them, have the right to refuse medical treatment.

III. DECISIONMAKING CAPACITY AND COMPETENCE

A proper determination of capacity is crucial to an ethical decisionmaking process. These Guidelines define decisionmaking capacity as: (a) the ability to comprehend information relevant to the decision; (b) the ability to deliberate about the choices in accordance with personal values and goals; and (c) the ability to communicate (verbally or nonverbally) with caregivers. Caregivers have a duty to respect the patient as a self-determining individual; they must consequently avoid wresting control from the patient with decisionmaking capacity. Caregivers also have a duty to protect the well-being of the patient; thus they must shield patients who lack decisionmaking capacity from the potentially harmful consequences of their own choices. Viewing capable patients as incapable, or viewing incapable patients as capable can both do serious harm.

There is considerable confusion about capacity. One source of difficulty is the widespread tendency to confuse the notions of "capacity" and "competence." A growing number of authorities have underscored the important distinction between these terms. "Competence" and "incompetence" should be understood as legal terms of art; their use should be restricted to situations in which a formal judicial determination has been made. Under the law, until such time as a judicial determination of incompetence has been made, individuals are presumed competent to manage their own affairs.

Decisionmaking capacity, as we elaborate below, refers to a patient's functional ability* to make informed health care decisions in accordance with personal values. Unlike a determination of competence, a determination of capacity is not a product of a judicial proceeding. A person can be legally competent and nonetheless lack the capacity to make a particular treatment decision. Conversely, a person who has been declared legally incompetent for other purposes (such as financial decisions) may still possess the capacity to make a treatment decision. Capacity or incapacity is also not a diagnostic category. A person can have a psychiatric disorder, or an organic mental disability such as mild retardation or dementia, and still have the functional capacity to make a particular decision. Finally, capacity is choice specific: a person may have the capacity to make one treatment choice but not another.

A second source of confusion is the lack of agreement on the appropriate standard to use in determining capacity. A number of different and competing standards have been proposed. The key alternatives are: (1) an *outcome standard* in which capacity is judged solely by the content and consequences of the patient's treatment choice; (2) a *status or category standard* in which all patients with certain characteristics (retarded people and minors, for example) are automatically judged to lack decisionmaking capacity; and (3) a *process standard* in which capacity is determined by assessing the patient's exercise of particular abilities in the decisionmaking process.

We believe that the process standard should be used in determining capacity. This standard is the most flexible and sensitive to each patient's circumstances, and strikes the most reasonable balance between the patient's autonomy and well-being. The outcome standard places too much weight on narrow medical criteria, and runs too great a risk of inappropriately denying the capacity of patients who make idiosyncratic choices to forgo life-sustaining treatment. The status or category standard would pose no problems if it applied only to obvious categories of patients without decisionmaking capacity such as unconscious persons; in such cases, however, it would not differ from assessments based on the process standard. But problems arise when it includes categories such as minors or retarded people. Individual variations exist within these classes of patients, and the categorical approach would be over-inclusive—determining that all lack capacity. The categorical approach also has significant potential for abuse in the

---

* This should not be confused with a different use of the term in geriatrics to mean the capacity to perform certain tasks, such as activities of daily living.

case of the elderly, and would invite the dangers inherent in all age-based classifications, as discussed in Section V, p. 135.

The process standard respects the patient's self-determination while protecting the patient from the harmful consequences of choices made without capacity. The more harmful to the patient his or her choice appears to be, the higher the level of capacity required and the greater the level of certainty the professional should have about the assessment of capacity. Decisions to forgo life-sustaining treatment vary substantially in their effects on the patient. When a decision ends a life of intolerable and irreversible suffering it may have a salutary effect; when it only affects the time of death by a very short period (such as a matter of hours), the effect may be negligible; when a treatment that could save life and restore function is refused, the effect may be very grave.

Capacity is not an all-or-nothing matter; there is a spectrum of abilities, and capacity can fluctuate over time and in different circumstances. (Fluctuating capacity should be distinguished from a fluctuating choice—a patient may have decisionmaking capacity even though the patient changes his or her mind. Extreme instability of preference, however, may itself be a form of decisionmaking incapacity.) Moreover, a patient's capacity need not be perfect or unaffected to be adequate for the decision at hand. Patients should be presumed to have capacity. They should be relieved of decisionmaking authority only when their level of capacity, or the caregiver's level of certainty about that capacity, is inadequate in light of the gravity of the consequences at stake.

In determining capacity, careful attention must be paid to the timing of the determination and the setting in which it is made. Professionals who make these determinations should be alert to numerous factors, such as temporary depression or the side effects of medication, that may affect the relevant functional abilities of the patient. They should take steps to alleviate conditions that produce incapacity before pursuing the avenues of surrogate decisionmaking outlined in the Guidelines. Even patients without capacity can often be helped to participate in the decisionmaking process, and this should be done whenever possible.

IV. "QUALITY OF LIFE"

Whether to consider the "quality of life" of patients when deciding about forgoing life-sustaining treatment is one of the major moral dilemmas of modern medicine. Medicine has developed the capacity to delay death, but the lives thus prolonged may not be worth living to some of these patients. Moreover, in making treatment decisions there is often a question of which choice will produce a better "quality of life" for the patient, but it is often not clear how to answer that question.

Some view the term "quality of life" as a euphemism for the judgment that certain individuals, who are in very poor condition, are valueless to society and ought to be allowed to die. That kind of a judgment would be unethical and we reject it; the ethical justification for sustaining a person's life is not determined by his or her worth to society. In contrast we consider "quality of life" to be an ethically essential concept that focuses on the good of the individual, what kind of life is possible given the person's condition, and whether that condition will allow the individual to have a life that he or she views as worth living. In this second sense, the life of an individual is evaluated not according to its worth to others, but according to its worth to the individual himself or herself. Even a person with a serious illness or extremely disabling condition can find satisfaction in life. There is no single "quality of life" experienced by all people with a certain condition. The satisfactions, joy, burdens, and suffering experienced vary tremendously from one person to the next.

When people with decisionmaking capacity make "quality of life" judgments to determine their own medical treatment preferences, that is generally accepted as ethically sound. In fact, patients and health care professionals make judgments about "quality of life" all the time outside of termination of treatment contexts. A common goal of various kinds of medical treatment (for example, rehabilitative care) is the enhancement of the patient's "quality of life." Indeed, health care professionals should always try to enhance the quality of a patient's life, as evaluated from the patient's perspective. When a surrogate or health care professional makes such a "quality of life" judgment instead of a patient, however, discomfort arises. It is all too easy for surrogates and professionals to project their own attitudes about "quality of life" onto the patient, either in applying the patient's own previously stated preferences and values to the treatment choice or in deciding what a reasonable person in the patient's circumstances would want.

Even if the surrogate and professional avoid this kind of projection, the question remains what relevance does "quality of life" have and what should it mean? Some people believe that we should consider the "quality of life" of persons without decisionmaking capacity even when we know nothing of the patient's treatment preferences and the patient's subjective experience of his or her condition. This risks adopting a "quality of life" standard in the sense of worth to society. Others maintain that "quality of life" judgments should simply not be made for persons who lack decisionmaking capacity; but a failure to do so may condemn some patients to lives of indignity, pain, or burden that no person with decisionmaking capacity would choose.

The best we can do in these circumstances is to allow individuals to choose for themselves before they become incapacitated, or allow their surrogates in consultation with health care professionals to choose as they would have wanted—as best we can know—after they lose decisionmaking capacity. At the same time, we must scrutinize surrogates' decisions and health care professionals' assessments in order to guard against their projecting their own attitudes about "quality of life" onto the patient.

By allowing patients and their surrogates to make choices that consider "quality of life," we diminish the risk of forcing lives of pain, indignity, or overwhelming burden on those who are helpless. By applying the patient's view of "quality of life" we also avoid denigrating the worth of individual human beings, and instead respect their values and beliefs.

V. AGE AS A FACTOR IN DECISIONMAKING

Regardless of their age, human beings who face decisions about life-sustaining treatment are uniquely vulnerable; they need special protections, respect, and consideration from others. Such persons are usually seriously ill, gravely burdened by the present circumstances of their existence, and dependent upon the good will of their family, friends, and caregivers. At such a time, stereotypes and social prejudices are particularly demeaning and dangerous; special caution must be taken to prevent these attitudes from influencing decisions to terminate treatment.

There is today no serious moral controversy about the notion that prejudice based on race, sex, religion, or ethnic origin should play no part in decisions about medical treatment. But what of age? Here disagreement and moral uncertainty remain widespread. Many have argued that the patient's age should be a factor in termination of treatment decisions. They usually maintain that age should weigh against aggressive treatment, although age-based considerations logically could also tilt the other way. This is a special concern because many patients who face decisions about life-sustaining treatment are elderly people, and demographic trends suggest that this will be increasingly the case.

Factoring age into decisionmaking, like using "quality of life" considerations as discussed above, is worrisome mainly in the context of surrogate decisionmaking. No doubt adults with decisionmaking capacity often take their own age into consideration in decisions about life-sustaining treatment. Some may feel they are "too young to die," others may feel that they have "lived long enough." Either way, there seems to be nothing inherently objectionable about this when individuals are making decisions about their own treatment.

But matters are considerably more complex when a surrogate must weigh the benefits and burdens of medical treatment on another's behalf. As we noted above in discussing "quality of life," it is easy for surrogates, and indeed health care professionals, to project their own attitudes—here about aging—onto the patient in making decisions. Yet even when they avoid this, the question of the relevance of age remains, since there may be a reasonable and objective—and not simply a prejudicial—link between a person's age and how beneficial or burdensome life-sustaining treatment might be.

In coping with these difficult issues, the following distinctions may be helpful. First, it is important to distinguish between age and functional ability. The effects of disease and individual biological variations are such that an older patient may be stronger and have a better prognosis than a younger patient with essentially the same life-threatening condition. For this reason age is at best a crude and imprecise factor to use in assessing a given patient's prognosis and the benefits and burdens of a given treatment.

In surrogate decisionmaking, age should always give way to a more clinically precise and individualized assessment of the patient's underlying physiological status. Age *per se* is not a morally relevant factor in assessing the quality of extended life for an individual. An extra year of life at age 85, say, is not inherently either more or less meaningful or beneficial than an extra year of life at age 55 or even 25. These judgments must be individualized to each patient. To ignore the particular circumstances and values of the patient and to make judgments based on age alone are to fall prey to precisely the kind of dehumanizing age prejudice that ethical decisionmaking must avoid.

Second, considerations of age may have a different status and significance in policy decisions concerning the allocation of resources and the development of new technologies than they do in clinical decisions concerning the treatment of an individual patient. In clinical decisionmaking, individualized judgments and assessments are almost always possible; health care professionals and surrogates can and should look beyond age to functional ability and to the patient's values and circumstances. In matters of health policy and the allocation of scarce resources this is not the case. Policies often have to be made in terms of more general criteria and classifications. There may be reasons for using age as a yardstick in making policy choices and allocation decisions.

VI. ACCOMMODATING RELIGIOUS VALUES AND BELIEFS

These Guidelines attempt to set out an ethical framework for termination of treatment decisions that is compatible with a wide variety of theological perspectives and religious beliefs. No set of Guidelines based solely on the traditions and doctrines of one particular faith could provide a generally acceptable direction for decisions in this area. Individuals who disagree about religious fundamentals may nonetheless come by different routes to embrace the practical recommendations and Guidelines we offer here.

We are aware, however, that these decisions have controversial theological implications. Contemporary medicine has placed into human hands a new measure of control over the timing and circumstances of death. How we use that power affects not only individuals and their families, but the moral and spiritual dimensions of our culture as a whole. It affects the meaning we assign to death and the value we assign to life. These matters are and always have been of central concern to religious communities. Some voices in these communities have forcefully called attention to the dangers inherent in using this relatively new power. We must seriously consider their warnings, even when we might disagree with them.

There is one fundamental warning that we wish to address here. It is the fear that the law and the emerging ethical consensus on decisions to forgo life-sustaining treatment may establish both a process and a practice that are not sufficiently sensitive to specific religious values and not sufficiently flexible to accommodate religious objections.

Termination of treatment decisions are agonizing in the best of circumstances, and not every person who is directly or indirectly involved in these decisions—patient, family members, physicians, nurses, administrators, and others—is equally comfortable with the outcome. But at several different levels we should accommodate special religious concerns. As explained below, we have attempted to include such provisions in these Guidelines.

First and foremost, the religious values and beliefs of the individual patient should be respected. The principal means of doing this is to protect the autonomy of the individual patient in the decisionmaking process. Patients with decisionmaking capacity are free to bring their own religious convictions to bear in making choices about their care, and they should receive any pastoral support and counseling they desire. (See PART ONE: Section (1) (b), p. 19, and Section (4) (a), p. 26.) The autonomy and religious beliefs of patients without decisionmaking capacity are respected when their surrogates and caregivers strive to make decisions in light of what they know of the patient's values—from advance directives or other available information. (See PART ONE: Section (4)(c), p. 27.)

Second, health care professionals should not have to carry out treatment decisions that violate their own religious convictions. The health care system should honor conscientious requests for reassignment. This entails administrative and institutional costs; but the moral integrity of health care professionals deserves respect. (See PART ONE: Section (8)(e), p. 32.)

At two places in the Guidelines, religious issues arise more specifically. PART TWO: Section B presents Guidelines on accommodating religious objections to the use of blood and blood products. The Guidelines recommend honoring religious refusals in most cases.

PART FOUR considers the tension between societal needs and religious beliefs in establishing criteria for declaring death. Some, on religious grounds, reject using neurological criteria for declaring death. This is one area where society's needs should take precedence over individual autonomy and religious liberty. Allowing religious minorities to exempt themselves from society's criteria for recognizing and declaring death would create confusion; some patients would be considered alive instead of dead simply because of particular religious convictions. Uniform criteria, including neurological criteria, are necessary. (See PART FOUR: Section (2), p. 88.)

There is a related problem that is more difficult to resolve. Some members of religious minorities who reject neurological criteria claim that if the patient is determined to be dead using neurological criteria, but circulatory and other physiological functions can be sustained for a period, it should be permissible to continue treatment if the responsible health care professional is willing. Others feel that this would be wasteful care or offensive to health care professionals. The nurses who would care for the body most intimately might feel particularly offended. In addition, the practice of allowing some dead bodies to be treated as if they were still alive, depending on the person's religion, could undermine confidence in the criteria for determining death.

This conflict is not resolved in the Guidelines. The Guidelines, however, do make the procedural recommendation that a hospital which chooses to allow the practice of continued treatment after a determination of death should solicit a range of views on the pertinent issues and adopt explicit policy. (See PART FOUR: Section (3), p. 89.) This will ensure that people are aware of the practice, become informed about the issues, and can debate them.

GLOSSARY

1. An **advance directive** is a document in which a person gives advance directions about medical care, or designates who should make medical decisions for the person if he or she should lose decision-making capacity, or both. There are two types of advance directives: treatment directives and proxy directives.

2. **Cardiopulmonary resuscitation** (CPR) is an array of interventions undertaken at the time of a cardiac or respiratory arrest to restore heartbeat and breathing.

3. A **"do not resuscitate"** (DNR) order is a signed order directing that no CPR efforts are to be undertaken in the event of a cardiac or respiratory arrest.

4. A **durable power of attorney** (DPA) is an individual's written designation of another person to act on his or her behalf, when the designation is authorized by a state's durable power of attorney statute. Under state law, a power of attorney terminates when the designating individual loses decisionmaking capacity, whereas a durable power of attorney does not. A DPA is one type of proxy directive.

5. An **emergency** is a sudden, acute medical crisis in the condition of a patient, requiring immediate medical attention in order to avoid injury, impairment, or death.

6. **Ethics** refers to principles of morality and of right and wrong conduct, as the term is used in these Guidelines. Although some scholars distinguish between ethics and morality, we make no distinction here.

7. **Hand feeding** is a procedure in which the patient is fed by another person who puts food into the patient's mouth, as by spoon or syringe.

8. **Health care personnel** are all persons involved in providing health care for patients. This includes both health care professionals and non-professional health care workers involved in patient care, such as nurses' aides.

9. A **health care professional** is a physician, nurse, or other professional who provides health care.

10. The **health care team** consists of all health care personnel involved in treating and caring for a particular patient.

11. A **life-sustaining treatment** is any medical intervention that is administered to a patient in order to prolong life and delay death.

12. For **"living will"** see "treatment directive."

13. **Medical** means pertaining to the treatment of diseases or pertaining to medicine as opposed to surgery, for the purposes of these Guidelines. It is not used here to refer to the concerns and practice of physicians as opposed to those of other health care professionals.

14. **Medical enteral procedures** are procedures in which nutritional formulas and water are introduced into the patient's stomach or intestine by means of a tube, such as a gastrostomy tube or nasogastric tube. The term "enteral procedures" is commonly taken to include both intake by mouth and intake by tube. However, for the purposes of these Guidelines "medical enteral procedures" refers only to intake by tube.

15. **Medical ethics** refers generically in these Guidelines to physician, nursing, and other health care ethics.

16. **Medical procedures for supplying nutrition and hydration** are medical enteral procedures and parenteral nutritional procedures as each is defined in this Glossary.

17. **Pain relief** is the symptomatic control of physical and other pain.

18. **Palliative care** refers to medical, surgical, and other interventions to alleviate suffering, discomfort, and dysfunction, whether physical or not, but not to cure.

19. **Parenteral nutritional procedures** are procedures in which nutritional formulas and water are introduced into the patient's body by means other than the gastrointestinal tract. Such procedures include total parenteral nutritional support (TPN),

in which a formula capable of maintaining the patient for prolonged periods is infused into a vein— usually a large, central vein in the patient's chest— and intravenous procedures in which water and/ or a formula supplying limited nutritional support is introduced into a peripheral vein.

20. A **proxy directive** is an individual's written designation of another person to act on behalf of the designating individual in the event he or she becomes incapable of making decisions.

21. The **responsible health care professional** is the health care professional with primary responsibility for directing an individual's medical treatment. Typically this is a physician. Sometimes it is a nurse, particularly in nursing homes and home health care settings. Much more rarely, another health care professional may play this role.

22. A **surrogate** is an individual whose role it is to make health care decisions for another person.

23. **Terminally ill** means having an incurable or irreversible condition that has a high probability of causing death within a relatively short time with or without treatment. For the purposes of these Guidelines that time is defined as one year.

24. A **treatment directive** is a written statement prepared by an individual directing what forms of medical treatment the individual wishes to receive or forgo should he or she be in stated medical conditions (such as irreversible unconsciousness, severe and irreversible dementia, or terminal illness) and lack decisionmaking capacity. A "living will" is one kind of treatment directive.

BIBLIOGRAPHY

The Bibliography to these Guidelines lists those sources that we have found to be especially useful or thought-provoking. We do not attempt to list all of the many articles, books, and other documents currently available on these topics.

We use the following abbreviations:

JAMA Journal of the American Medical Association
NEJM New England Journal of Medicine

INTRODUCTION

Tom L. Beauchamp and James F. Childress, *Principles of Biomedical Ethics*, 2nd ed., New York: Oxford University Press, 1983.

Tom L. Beauchamp and Seymour Perlin, *Ethical Issues in Death & Dying*, Englewood Cliffs, N.J.: Prentice Hall, 1977.

Sissela Bok, Ethical Views, Part II of Death and Dying: Euthanasia and Sustaining Life: Ethical Views, in *Encyclopedia of Bioethics*, Vol. I, New York: The Free Press, 1978, pp. 268-278.

Daniel Callahan, Autonomy: A Moral Good, Not a Moral Obsession, 14 Hastings Center Report 40-42 (Oct. 1984).

Alexander M. Capron, Right to Refuse Medical Care, in *Encyclopedia of Bioethics*, Vol. I, New York: The Free Press, 1978, pp. 1498-1507.

Eric J. Cassell, Clinical Practice, Clinical Ethics (editorial), 145 Archives of Internal Medicine 627-628 (1985).

A. Edward Doudera and J. Douglas Peters, eds., *Legal and Ethical Aspects of Treating Critically and Terminally Ill Patients*, Ann Arbor: AUPHA Press, 1982.

Walter T. Eccard, A Revolution in White: New Approaches in Treating Nurses as Professionals, in Mathy D. Mezey and Diane O. McGivern, eds., *Nurses, Nurse Practitioners: The Evolution of Primary Care*, Boston: Little, Brown, 1986, pp. 380-405.

Ruth Faden and Tom Beauchamp, *History and Theory of Informed Consent*, New York: Oxford University Press, 1986.

Marvin Kohl, ed., *Beneficent Euthanasia*, Buffalo: Prometheus Books, 1975.

Jane Kummerer, Life Care Community Practice, in Mathy D. Mezey and Diane O. McGivern, eds., *Nurses, Nurse Practitioners: The Evolution of Primary Care*, Boston: Little, Brown, 1986, pp. 146-153.

Kevin D. O'Rourke and Dennis Brodeur, *Medical Ethics: Common Ground for Understanding*, St. Louis: The Catholic Health Association of the United States, 1986.

President's Commission for the Study of Ethical Problems in Medicine and Biomedical and Behavioral Research [hereinafter "President's Commission"], *Deciding to Forego Life-Sustaining Treatment: Ethical, Medical and Legal Issues in Treatment Decisions*, Washington, DC: U.S. Government Printing Office, 1983.

——————, *Making Health Care Decisions: The Ethical and Legal Implications of Informed Consent in the Patient-Practitioner Relationship*, Vol. I, Washington, DC: U.S. Government Printing Office, 1982.

Paul Ramsey, *Ethics at the Edges of Life*, New Haven: Yale University Press, 1978.

Bonnie Steinbock, ed., *Killing and Letting Die*, Englewood Cliffs, NJ: Prentice Hall, 1980.

Joyce B. Thompson and Henry O. Thompson, *Ethics in Nursing*, New York: Macmillan, 1981.

U.S. Congress, Office of Technology Assessment, *Life-Sustaining Technologies and the Elderly*, Washington, DC: U.S. Government Printing Office, 1987.

U.S. Congress, Office of Technology Assessment, *Nurse Practitioners, Physician Assistants, and Certified Nurse-Midwives: A Policy Analysis*, Health Technology Case Study 35, OTA-HCS-37, Washington, DC: U.S. Government Printing Office, 1986.

Robert M. Veatch, *Death, Dying, and the Biological Revolution: Our Last Quest for Responsibility*, New Haven: Yale University Press, 1976.

——————, ed., *Life Span: Values and Life-Extending Technologies*, San Francisco: Harper & Row, 1979.

Douglas N. Walton, *The Ethics of Withdrawal of Life-Supporting Systems: Case Studies on Decision-Making in Intensive Care*, Westport, CT: Greenwood Press, 1983.

PART ONE: Making Treatment Decisions — Guidelines on the Decisionmaking Process

American Nurses' Association, *Perspectives on the Code for Nurses*, 1978.

Richard W. Besdine, Decisions to Withhold Treatment from Nursing Home Residents, 31 Journal of the American Geriatrics Society 602-606 (1983).

Eric J. Cassell, Autonomy in the Intensive Care Unit: The Refusal of Treatment, in James P. Orlowski and George Kanote, eds., *Critical Care Clinics: Ethical Moments in Critical Care Medicine*, Vol. II, Philadelphia: W. B. Saunders Co., 1986, pp. 27-40.

——————, *Talking With Patients*, Vol. II, *Clinical Technique*, Cambridge: MIT Press, 1985, Ch. 5.

Joan Lynaugh, Narrow Passageways: Nurses and Physicians in Conflict and Concert Since 1875, in Tristram Englehardt and Stuart Spicker, eds., *The Physician as Captain of the Ship: A Critical Reappraisal*, Boston: D. Reidel, forthcoming 1987.

D. Joanne Lynn, Deciding about Life-Sustaining Treatment, in Christine K. Cassel and John R. Walsh, eds., *Geriatric Medicine*, Vol. II, *Fundamentals of Geriatric Care*, New York: Springer Verlag, 1984, pp. 325-331.

——————, Dying and Dementia (editorial), 256 JAMA 2244-2245 (1986).

——————, Ethical Issues in Caring for Elderly Residents of Nursing Homes, 13 Primary Care 295-306 (1986).

Alan Meisel et al., Hospital Guidelines for Deciding about Life-Sustaining Treatment: Dealing with Health Limbo, 14 Critical Care Medicine 239-246 (1986).

Alan Meisel and Lisa D. Kabnick, Informed Consent to Medical Treatment: An Analysis of Recent Legislation, 41 University of Pittsburgh Law Review 407-564 (1980).

Barbara Mishkin, *A Matter of Choice: Planning Ahead for Health Care Decisions,* Washington, DC: American Association of Retired Persons, 1986.

President's Commission, *Deciding to Forego Life-Sustaining Treatment: Ethical, Medical and Legal Issues in Treatment Decisions*, Washington, DC: U.S. Government Printing Office, 1983.

——————, *Making Health Care Decisions: The Ethical and Legal Implications of Informed Consent in the Patient-Practitioner Relationship*, Vol. I, Washington, DC: U.S. Government Printing Office, 1982.

Nicholas Rango, The Nursing Home Resident with Dementia, 102 Annals of Internal Medicine 835-841 (1985).

E. Charlotte Theis, Ethical Issues: A Nursing Perspective, 315 NEJM 1222-1224 (1986).

Robert M. Veatch, Limits of Guardian Treatment Refusal: A Reasonableness Standard, 9 American Journal of Law and Medicine 427-468 (1984).

——————, Nursing Ethics, Physician Ethics, and Medical Ethics, 9 Law, Medicine and Health Care 17-19 (Oct. 1981).

Sidney H. Wanzer et al., The Physician's Responsibility Toward Hopelessly Ill Patients, 310 NEJM 955-959 (1984).

PART TWO: Specific Treatment Modalities

A. Guidelines on Long-Term Life-Supporting Technology — Ventilators and Dialysis

Ventilators:

Ned H. Cassem, When to Disconnect the Respirator, 9 Psychiatric Annals 38-53 (1979).

Ake Grenvik, Terminal Weaning: Discontinuance of Life-Supporting Therapy in the Terminally Ill Patient (editorial), 11 Critical Care Medicine 394-395 (1983).

Dialysis:

James D. Campbell and Anne R. Campbell, The Social and Economic Costs of End-Stage Renal Disease: A Patient's Perspective, 299 NEJM 386-392 (1978).

Roger W. Evans et al., The Quality of Life of Patients with End-Stage Renal Disease, 312 NEJM 553-559 (1985).

Renée C. Fox and Judith P. Swazey, *The Courage to Fail: A Social View of Organ Transplants and Dialysis*, 2nd ed., Chicago: University of Chicago Press, 1978.

Jay Katz and Alexander M. Capron, *Catastrophic Diseases: Who Decides What? A Psychosocial and*

Legal Analysis of the Problems Posed by Hemodialysis and Organ Transplantation, New York: Russell Sage Foundation, 1975.

Gina Bari Kolata, Dialysis After Nearly a Decade, 208 Science 473-476 (1980).

Steven Neu and Carl M. Knellstrand, Stopping Long-Term Dialysis: An Empirical Study of Withdrawal of Life-Supporting Treatment, 314 NEJM 14-20 (1986).

Drummond Rennie, Renal Rehabilitation — Where are the Data?, 304 NEJM 351-352 (1981).

B. Guidelines on Emergency Interventions — Cardiopulmonary Resuscitation (CPR) and Treatment for Life-Threatening Bleeding

Cardiopulmonary Resuscitation:

Marcia Angell, Respecting the Autonomy of Competent Patients (editorial), 310 NEJM 1115-1116 (1984).

Susanna E. Bedell et al., Survival after Cardiopulmonary Resuscitation in the Hospital, 309 NEJM 569-576 (1983).

Susanna E. Bedell and Thomas L. Delbanco, Choices About Cardiopulmonary Resuscitation in the Hospital: When Do Physicians Talk with Patients?, 310 NEJM 1089-1093 (1984).

Andrew L. Evans and Baruch A. Brody, The Do-Not-Resuscitate Order in Teaching Hospitals, 253 JAMA 2236-2239 (1985).

Neil J. Farber et al., Cardiopulmonary Resuscitation (CPR), Patient Factors and Decision Making, 144 Archives of Internal Medicine 2229-2232 (1984).

Maurice Fox and Helena Levens Lipton, The Decision to Perform Cardiopulmonary Resuscitation (editorial), 309 NEJM 607-608 (1983).

Joint Commission on Accreditation of Hospitals, Do Not Resuscitate Standards Sent for Field Review, 7 JCAH Perspectives 4 (Jan./Feb. 1987).

Melinda A. Lee and Christine K. Cassell, The Ethical and Legal Framework for the Decision Not To Resuscitate, 140 Western Journal of Medicine 117-122 (1984).

Helene L. Lipton, Do-Not-Resuscitate Decisions in a Community Hospital, 256 JAMA 1164-1169 (1986).

Bernard Lo et al., "Do Not Resuscitate" Decisions: A Prospective Study at Three Teaching Hospitals, 145 Archives of Internal Medicine 1115-1117

(1985).

Steven H. Miles et al., The Do-Not-Resuscitate Order in a Teaching Hospital: Considerations and a Suggested Policy, 96 Annals of Internal Medicine 660-664 (1982).

Mitchell T. Rabkin et al., Orders Not To Resuscitate, 295 NEJM 364-366 (1976).

Richard F. Uhlmann et al., Epidemiology of No-Code Orders in an Academic Hospital, 140 Western Journal of Medicine 114-116 (1984).

Robert M. Veatch, Deciding Against Resuscitation: Encouraging Signs and Potential Dangers (editorial), 253 JAMA 77-78 (1985).

Arnold Wagner, Cardiopulmonary Resuscitation in the Aged: A Prospective Survey, 310 NEJM 1129-1130 (1984).

Stuart J. Younger et al., "Do Not Resuscitate" Orders: Incidence and Implications in a Medical Intensive Care Unit, 253 JAMA 54-57 (1985).

Bleeding:

N. C. Drew, The Pregnant Jehovah's Witness, 7 Journal of Medical Ethics 137-139 (Sept. 1981).

Larry J. Findley and Paul M. Redstone, Blood Transfusion in Adult Jehovah's Witnesses: A Case Study of One Congregation, 142 Archives of Internal Medicine 606-607 (1982).

Medical Department, World Headquarters of Jehovah's Witnesses, Professionally Speaking: Refusal of Blood — An Ethical Issue?, 246 JAMA 2471-2472 (1981).

Note, Their Life is in the Blood: Jehovah's Witnesses, Blood Transfusions and the Courts, 10 Northern Kentucky Law Review 281-304 (1983).

Total Exsanguination After Refusal of Blood Transfusion (letters), 306 NEJM 544-545 (1982).

C. Guidelines on Medical Procedures for Supplying Nutrition and Hydration

George J. Annas, Do Feeding Tubes Have More Rights Than Patients?, 16 Hastings Center Report 26-28 (Feb. 1986).

——————, Nonfeeding: Lawful Killing in CA, Homicide in NJ, 13 Hastings Center Report 19-20 (Dec. 1983).

Daniel Callahan, On Feeding the Dying, 13 Hastings Center Report 22-27 (Oct. 1983).

Alexander M. Capron, Ironies and Tensions in

Feeding the Dying, 14 Hastings Center Report 32-35 (Oct. 1984).

Eric J. Cassell, Life as a Work of Art, 14 Hastings Center Report 35-37 (Oct. 1984).

Patrick G. Derr, Why Food and Fluids Can Never be Denied, 16 Hastings Center Report 28-30 (Feb. 1986).

Willard Green, Setting Boundaries for Artificial Feeding, 14 Hastings Center Report 8-11 (Dec. 1984).

Dorothy G. King and Julie O'Sullivan Maillet, Position of the American Dietetic Association: Issues in Feeding the Terminally Ill Adult, 87 Journal of the American Dietetic Association 78-85 (Jan. 1987).

Bernard Lo and Laurie Dornbrand, Guiding the Hand that Feeds: Caring for the Demented Elderly, 311 NEJM 402-404 (1984).

Joanne Lynn, ed., *By No Extraordinary Means*, Bloomington: Indiana University Press, 1986.

Joanne Lynn and James F. Childress, Must Patients Always be Given Food and Water?, 13 Hastings Center Report 17-21 (Oct. 1983).

Gilbert Meilaender, On Removing Food and Water: Against the Stream, 14 Hastings Center Report ll-13 (Dec. 1984).

Kenneth C. Micetich et al., Are Intravenous Fluids Morally Required for a Dying Patient?, 143 Archives of Internal Medicine 975-978 (1983).

Steven H. Miles, The Terminally Ill Elderly: Dealing with the Ethics of Feeding, 40 Geriatrics 112-120 (1985).

Kevin O'Rourke, The A.M.A. Statement on Tube Feeding: An Ethical Analysis, 155 America 321-323, 331 (1986).

John J. Paris, When Burdens of Feeding Outweigh Benefits, 16 Hastings Center Report 30-32 (Feb. 1986).

John J. Paris and Anne Fletcher, Infant Doe Regulations and the Absolute Requirement to Use Nourishment and Fluids for the Dying Patient, 11 Law, Medicine and Health Care 210-213 (1983).

Mark Siegler and Alan J. Weisbard, Against the Emerging Stream: Should Fluids and Nutritional Support Be Discontinued?, 145 Archives of Internal Medicine 129-131 (1985).

Joyce V. Zerwekh, The Dehydration Question, 83 Nursing 17-19 (1983).

D. Guidelines on Antibiotics and Other Life-Sustaining Medication

Norman K. Brown and Donovan J. Thompson, Nontreatment of Fever in Extended Care Facilities, 300 NEJM 1246-1250 (1979).

Richard A. Garibaldi et al., Infections Among Patients in Nursing Homes: Policies, Prevalence and Problems, 305 NEJM 731-735 (1981).

Richard A. Gleckman and Nelson M. Gantz, eds., *Infections in the Elderly*, Boston: Little, Brown, 1983.

David Hilfiker, Allowing the Debilitated to Die: Facing our Ethical Choices, 308 NEJM 716-719 (1983).

Edward W. Hook et al., Failure of Intensive Care Unit Support to Influence Mortality from Pneumococcal Bacteremia, 249 JAMA 1055-1057 (1983).

Sidney H. Wanzer et al., The Physician's Responsibility Toward Hopelessly Ill Patients, 310 NEJM 955-959 (1984).

E. Guidelines on Palliative Care and the Relief of Pain

Marcia Angell, The Quality of Mercy (editorial), 306 NEJM 98-99 (1982).

John J. Bonica and Vittorio Ventafridda, eds., *International Symposium on Pain of Advanced Cancer, Advances in Pain Research Therapy*, Vol. II, New York: Raven Press, 1979.

Eric J. Cassell, The Relief of Suffering, 143 Archives of Internal Medicine 522-523 (1983).

Maureen Cushing, Cause of Death: Drug or Disease?, 83 American Journal of Nursing 943-944 (1983).

Kathleen M. Foley, The Treatment of Cancer Pain, 313 NEJM 84-95 (1985).

Joanne Lynn, Care Near the End of Life, in Christine K. Cassel and John R. Walsh, eds., *Geriatric Medicine*, Vol. II, *Fundamentals of Geriatric Care*, New York: Springer Verlag, 1984, pp. 332-343.

Joanne Lynn, Legal and Ethical Issues in Palliative Health Care, 12 Seminars in Oncology 476-481 (1985).

Ronald Malzack, *The Challenge of Pain*, New York: Basic Books, 1982.

Richard M. Marks and Edward J. Sachar, Undertreatment of Medical Inpatients with Narcotic Analgesics, 78 Annals of Internal Medicine 173-

181 (1973).

Jane Porter and Hershel Jick, Addiction Rare in Patients Treated with Narcotics (letter), 302 NEJM 123 (1980).

Marcus Reidenberg, ed., Symposium on Clinical Pharmacology of Symptom Control, 66 Medical Clinics of North America 969-1187 (1982).

Cicely M. Saunders, ed., *The Management of Terminal Disease*, London: Edward Arnold, 1978.

The Task Force on Supportive Care, The Supportive Care Plan — Its Meaning and Application: Recommendations and Guidelines, 12 Law, Medicine and Health Care 97-102 (June 1984).

D.W. Vere, The Hospital as a Place of Pain, 6 Journal of Medical Ethics 117-119 (1980).

PART THREE: Prospective Planning—Guidelines on Advance Directives

Sissela Bok, Personal Directions for Care at the End of Life, 295 NEJM 367-369 (1976).

Stuart J. Eisendrath and Albert R. Jonsen, The Living Will: Help or Hindrance?, 249 JAMA 2054-2058 (1983).

Steven A. Levenson et al., Ethical Considerations in Critical and Terminal Illness in the Elderly, 29 Journal of the American Geriatrics Society 563-567 (1981).

Joanne Lynn, Availability of Durable Power of Attorney for Health Care (letter), 312 NEJM 248 (1985).

Steven H. Miles, Advance Directives to Limit Treatment: The Need for Portability, 35 Journal of the American Geriatrics Society 74-76 (1987).

President's Commission, *Deciding to Forego Life-Sustaining Treatment: Ethical, Medical, and Legal Issues in Treatment Decisions*, Washington, DC: U.S. Government Printing Office, 1983.

Arnold S. Relman, Michigan's Sensible "Living Will," 300 NEJM 1270-1271 (1979).

Society for the Right to Die, *Handbook of 1985 Living Will Laws*, New York: Society for the Right to Die, 1986.

Robert Steinbrook et al., Preferences of Homosexual Men with AIDS for Life-Sustaining Treatment, 314 NEJM 457-460 (1986).

Robert Steinbrook and Bernard Lo, Decision Making for Incompetent Patients by Designated Proxy: California's New Law, 310 NEJM 1598-1601
(1984).

PART FOUR: Declaring Death — Guidelines on the Declaration of Death

Ad Hoc Committee of the Harvard Medical School to Examine the Definition of Brain Death, A Definition of Irreversible Coma, 205 JAMA 337-340 (1968).

Alexander M. Capron and Leon R. Kass, A Statutory Definition of the Standards for Determining Human Death: An Appraisal and a Proposal, 21 University of Pennsylvania Law Review 87-118 (1972).

Alexander M. Capron and Joanne Lynn, Defining Death (letter), 215 Science 612 (1982).

Ronald E. Cranford and Harmon L. Smith, Some Critical Distinctions Between Brain Death and the Persistent Vegetative State, 6 Ethics in Science and Medicine 199-209 (1979).

Ake Grenvik et al., Cessation of Therapy in Terminal Illness and Brain Death, 6 Critical Care Medicine 284-291 (1978).

Joanne Lynn, Diagnosis of Brain Death (letter), 250 JAMA 612-613 (1983).

——————, The Determination of Death, 99 Annals of Internal Medicine 264-266 (1983).

New York State Task Force on Life and the Law, *The Determination of Death*, New York, 1986.

President's Commission, *Defining Death: Medical, Legal and Ethical Issues in the Determination of Death*, Washington, DC: U.S. Government Printing Office, 1981.

A Report by the Task Force on Death and Dying of the Institute of Society, Ethics and the Life Sciences [The Hastings Center], Requirements for the Determination of Death: An Appraisal, 221 JAMA 48-53 (1972).

Robert M. Veatch, The Definition of Death: Ethical, Philosophical, and Policy Confusion, 315 Annals of the New York Academy of Science 307-321 (1978).

PART FIVE: Policy Considerations

A. Guidelines on Ethics Committees

Cynthia B. Cohen, Interdisciplinary Consultation on Care of the Critically Ill and Dying: The Role of One Hospital Ethics Committee, 10 Critical

Care Medicine 776-784 (1982).

Ronald E. Cranford et al., Institutional Ethics Committees: Issues of Confidentiality and Immunity, 13 Law, Medicine and Health Care 52-60 (Apr. 1985).

Ronald E. Cranford and A. Edward Doudera, The Emergence of Institutional Ethics Committees, 12 Law, Medicine and Health Care 13-20 (Feb. 1984).

_____ and _____, eds., *Institutional Ethics Committees and Health Care Decision Making*, Ann Arbor: Health Administration Press, 1984.

Ronald E. Cranford and John C. Roberts, Biomedical Ethics Committees, 13 Primary Care 327-341 (1986).

Kathleen Esqueda, Hospital Ethics Committees: Four Case Studies, 7 Hospital Medical Staff 26-31 (1978).

Bowen Hosford, *Bioethics Committees*, Rockville, MD: Aspen Systems Corporation, 1986.

Geanie Schmit Kayser-Jones, Distributive Justice and the Treatment of Active Illness in Nursing Homes, 23 Social Science and Medicine 1279-1286 (1987).

Carol Levine, Hospital Ethics Committees: A Guarded Prognosis, 7 Hastings Center Report 25-27 (June 1977).

Richard A. McCormick, Ethics Committees: Promise or Peril?, 12 Law, Medicine and Health Care 150-155 (Sept. 1984).

President's Commission, *Deciding to Forego Life-Sustaining Treatment: Ethical, Medical and Legal Issues in Treatment Decisions*, Washington, DC: U.S. Government Printing Office, 1983.

_____, *Making Health Care Decisions: The Ethical and Legal Implications of Informed Consent in the Patient-Practitioner Relationship*, Vol. I, Washington, DC: U.S. Government Printing Office, 1982.

John A. Robertson, Ethics Committees in Hospitals: Alternative Structures and Responsibilities, 10 Quality Review Bulletin 6-10 (Jan. 1984).

Mark Siegler, Ethics Committees: Decisions by Bureaucracy, 16 Hastings Center Report 22-24 (June 1986).

Karen Teel, The Physician's Dilemma — A Doctor's View: What the Law Should Be, 27 Baylor Law Review 6-9 (1975).

Robert M. Veatch, Hospital Ethics Committees: Is There a Role?, 7 Hastings Center Report 22-

25 (June 1977).

Susan M. Wolf, Ethics Committees in the Courts, 16 Hastings Center Report 12-15 (June 1986).

B. Guidelines on Institutional Policies for Patient Admissions and Transfers

H. Tristam Englehardt, Jr. and Michael A. Rie, Intensive Care Units, Scarce Resources, and Conflicting Principles of Justice, 255 JAMA 1159-1164 (1986).

Susan Dadakis Horn, Measuring Severity of Illness: Comparisons Across Institutions, 73 American Journal of Public Health 25-31 (1983).

William A. Knaus et al., APACHE—Acute Physiology and Chronic Health Evaluation: A Physiologically Based Classification System, 9 Critical Care Medicine 591-597 (1981).

William A. Knaus and George E. Thibault, Intensive Care Units Today, in Barbara J. McNeil and Ernest G. Cravalho, eds., *Critical Issues in Medical Technology*, Boston: Auburn House, 1982, pp. 193-215.

Stuart E. Lind, Transferring the Terminally Ill, 311 NEJM 1181-1182 (1984).

Joanne Lynn, Ethics in Hospice Care, in Lenora Finn Paradis, ed., *Hospice Handbook: A Guide for Managers*, Rockville, MD: Aspen Systems, 1985, pp. 303-324.

Henry S. Perkins et al., Providers as Predictors: Using Outcome Predictions in Intensive Care, 14 Critical Care Medicine 105-110 (1986).

Bruce E. Zawacki, ICU Physician's Ethical Role in Distributing Scarce Resources, 13 Critical Care Medicine 57-60 (1985).

C. The Use of Economic Considerations in Decisions Concerning Life-Sustaining Treatments

Henry J. Aaron and William B. Schwartz, *The Painful Prescription: Rationing Hospital Care*, Washington, DC: Brookings Institution, 1984.

Marcia Angell, Cost Containment and the Physician, 254 JAMA 1203-1207 (1985).

Jerome L. Avorn, Benefit and Cost Analysis in Geriatric Care, Turning Age Discrimination into Health Policy, 310 NEJM 1294-1301 (1984).

Ronald Bayer et al., The Care of the Terminally Ill: Morality and Economics, 309 NEJM 1490-

1494 (1983).

Joesph F. Boyle, Should We Learn to Say No?, 252 JAMA 782-784 (1984).

Dan W. Brock and Allen Buchanan, Ethical Issues in For-Profit Health Care, in Bradford H. Gray, ed., *For-Profit Enterprise in Health Care*, Washington, DC: National Academy Press, 1986, pp. 224-249.

John P. Bunker, When Doctors Disagree, The New York Review of Books 7-12 (Apr. 25, 1985).

Norman Daniels, Why Saying No to Patients in the United States Is So Hard: Cost Containment, Justice, and Provider Autonomy, 314 NEJM 1380-1383 (1986).

H. Tristram Englehardt, Jr. and Michael A. Rie, Intensive Care Units, Scarce Resources, and Conflicting Principles of Justice, 255 JAMA 1159-1164 (1986).

Roger W. Evans, Health Care Technology and the Inevitability of Resource Allocation and Rationing Decisions, Part I, 249 JAMA 2047-2053, Part II, 249 JAMA 2208-2219 (1983).

Victor Fuchs, *The Health Economy*, Cambridge: Harvard University Press, 1986.

Eli Ginzberg, The Monetarization of Medical Care, 310 NEJM 1162-1165 (1984).

John K. Iglehart, Medical Care of the Poor — A Growing Problem, 313 NEJM 59-63 (1985).

Dana E. Johnson, Life, Death, and the Dollar Sign: Medical Ethics and Cost Containment, 252 JAMA 223-224 (1984).

Alexander Leaf, The Doctor's Dilemma — And Society's Too, 310 NEJM 718-720 (1984).

Walter J. McNerney, Control of Health-Care Costs in the 1980's, 303 NEJM 1088-1095 (1980).

David Mechanic, *From Advocacy to Allocation: The Evolving American Health Care System*, New York: The Free Press, 1986.

Paul T. Menzel, *Medical Costs, Moral Choices: A Philosophy of Health Care Economics in America*, New Haven: Yale University Press, 1983.

Mary O'Neil Mundinger, Health Service Funding Cuts and the Declining Health of the Poor, 313 NEJM 44-47 (1985).

Edmund D. Pellegrino, Rationing Health Care: The Ethics of Medical Gatekeeping, 2 Journal of Contemporary Health, Law and Policy 23-45 (1986).

Roger Platt, Cost Containment — Another View, 309 NEJM 726-730 (1983).

President's Commission, *Securing Access to Health Care: The Ethical Implications of Differences in the Availability of Health Services*, Vol. I, Washington, DC: U.S. Government Printing Office, 1983.

Arnold S. Relman, Economic Considerations in Emergency Care: What Are Hospitals For?, 312 NEJM 372-373 (1985).

Carl J. Schramm, Can We Solve the Hospital-Cost Problem in Our Democracy?, 311 NEJM 729-732 (1984).

Steven A. Schroeder, Doctors and the Medical Cost Crisis: Culprits, Victims, or Solution?, 48 The Pharos 12-18 (Spring 1985).

Anne A. Scitovsky, "The High Cost of Dying": What Do the Data Show?, 62 Milbank Memorial Fund Quarterly 591-608 (1984).

Anne A. Scitovsky and Alexander M. Capron, Medical Care at the End of Life: The Interaction of Economics and Ethics, 7 Annual Review of Public Health 59-75 (1986).

Jonathan A. Showstack et al., The Role of Changing Clinical Practices in the Rising Costs of Hospital Care, 313 NEJM 1201-1208 (1985).

Lester C. Thurow, Medicine Versus Economics, 313 NEJM 611-614 (1985).

Robert M. Veatch, DRGs and the Ethical Allocation of Resources, 16 Hastings Center Report 32-40 (June 1986).

PART SIX: Special Problems

I. Terminating Treatment, Active Voluntary Euthanasia, and Assisting Suicide

Jonathan Bennett, Morality and Consequences, *The Tanner Lectures on Human Values*, Vol. II, Salt Lake City: University of Utah Press, 1981.

—————, Whatever the Consequences, 26 Analysis 83-102 (1966).

Joseph Boyle, On Killing and Letting Die, 51 New Scholasticism 433-452 (1977).

Dan W. Brock, Taking Human Life, 95 Ethics 851-865 (1985).

K. Danner Clouser, Allowing or Causing: Another Look, 87 Annals of Internal Medicine 622-624 (1977).

Daniel Dinello, On Killing and Letting Die, 31 Analysis 84-86 (1971).

Matthew Edlund and Laurence R. Tancredi, Quality of Life: An Ideological Critique, 28 Perspectives in Biology and Medicine 591-607 (1985).

Philippa Foot, Euthanasia, 6 Philosophy and Public Affairs 85-112 (1977).

Jonathan Glover, *Causing Death and Saving Lives*, Middlesex, England: Penguin Books, 1977.

H.L. Hart and Tony Honore, *Causation in the Law*, 2nd ed., Oxford: Oxford University Press, 1969.

Dennis Horan and David Mall, *Death, Dying and Euthanasia*, Washington, DC: University Publications of America, 1977.

Yale Kamisar, Some Nonreligious Views Against Proposed "Mercy-Killing" Legislation, 42 Minnesota Law Review 969-1042 (1958).

Frances Kamm, Killing and Letting Die: Methodological and Substantive Issues, 64 Pacific Philosophical Quarterly 297-312 (1983).

Marvin Kohl, ed., *Beneficent Euthanasia*, Buffalo, NY: Prometheus Books, 1975.

John Ladd, ed., *Ethical Issues Relating to Life and Death*, New York: Oxford University Press, 1979.

Law Reform Commission of Canada, *Euthanasia, Aiding Suicide, and Cessation of Treatment*, Working Paper 28, Ottawa, 1982.

President's Commission, *Deciding to Forego Life-Sustaining Treatment: Ethical, Medical, and Legal Issues in Treatment Decisions*, Washington, DC: U.S. Government Printing Office, 1983.

James Rachels, *The End of Life: Euthanasia and Morality*, New York: Oxford University Press, 1986.

Bonnie Steinbock, ed., *Killing and Letting Die*, Englewood Cliffs, NJ: Prentice Hall, 1980.

Robert M. Veatch, *A Theory of Medical Ethics*, New York: Basic Books, 1981.

Douglas Walton, Omitting, Refraining and Letting Happen, 17 American Philosophical Quarterly 319-326 (1980).

II. Withholding and Withdrawing Treatment

President's Commission, *Deciding to Forego Life-Sustaining Treatment: Ethical, Medical, and Legal Issues in Treatment Desicions*, Washington, DC: U.S. Government Printing Office, 1983.

Paul Ramsey, *The Patient as Person*, New Haven: Yale University Press, 1976.

Douglas Walton, *Physician-Patient Decision-Making: A Study in Medical Ethics*, Westport,

CT: Greenwood Press, 1985.

III. Decisionmaking Capacity and Competence

Paul S. Appelbaum and Loren H. Roth, Clinical Issues in the Assessment of Competency, 138 American Journal of Psychiatry 1462-1467 (1981).

Willard Gaylin and Ruth Macklin, eds., *Who Speaks for the Child: The Problems of Proxy Consent*, New York: Plenum Press, 1982.

Alan Meisel, The "Exceptions" to the Informed Consent Doctrine: Striking a Balance Between Competing Values in Medical Decision-Making, 1979 Wisconsin Law Review 413-88 (1979).

President's Commission, *Making Health Care Decisions: The Ethical and Legal Implications of Informed Consent in the Patient-Practitioner Relationship*, Vol. I, Washington, DC: U.S. Government Printing Office, 1981.

Loren H. Roth et al., Tests of Competency to Consent to Treatment, 134 American Journal of Psychiatry 279-285 (1977).

Daniel Wikler, Paternalism and the Mildly Retarded, 8 Philosophy and Public Affairs 377-32 (Summer 1979).

IV. "Quality of Life"

George J. Annas, Quality of Life in the Courts: Earle Spring in Fantasyland, 10 Hastings Center Report 9-10 (Aug. 1980).

Michael Bayles, Euthanasia and the Quality of Life, in Michael D. Bayles and Dallas M. High, eds., *Medical Treatment of the Dying: Moral Issues*, Cambridge, MA: Schenkman Publishing Co., 1978, pp. 128-152.

Susan Braithwaite and David C. Thomasma, New Guidelines on Foregoing Life-Sustaining Treatment in Incompetent Patients: An Anticruelty Policy, 104 Annals of Internal Medicine 711-715 (1986).

Cynthia B. Cohen, "Quality of Life" and the Analogy with the Nazis, 8 Journal of Medicine and Philosophy 113-135 (1983).

Dallas High, Quality of Life and the Care of the Dying Person, in Michael D. Bayles and Dallas M. High, eds., *Medical Treatment of the Dying: Moral Issues*, Cambridge, MA: Schenkman Publishing Co., 1978, pp. 85-104.

Albert R. Jonsen et al., *Clinical Ethics*, New York:

Macmillan, 1982.

Edward W. Keyserlingk, *Sanctity of Life or Quality of Life, in the Context of Ethics, Medicine and Law*, Study Paper for the Law Reform Commission of Canada, Ottawa, 1979.

Richard A. McCormick, The Quality of Life, The Sanctity of Life, 8 Hastings Center Report 30-36 (Feb. 1978).

Robert A. Pearlman and Albert Jonsen, The Use of Quality-of-Life Considerations in Medical Decision Making, 33 Journal of the American Geriatrics Society 344-350 (1985).

Paul Ramsey, *Ethics at the Edges of Life*, New Haven: Yale University Press, 1978.

David C. Thomasma, Ethical Judgments of Quality of Life in the Care of the Aged, 32 Journal of the American Geriatrics Society 525-527 (1984).

V. Age as a Factor in Decisionmaking

Jerome L. Avorn, Benefit and Cost Analysis in Geriatric Care: Turning Age Discrimination into Health Policy, 310 NEJM 1294-1301 (1984).

Margaret P. Battin, Age Rationing and the Just Distribution of Health Care: Is There a Duty to Die?, 97 Ethics 317-340 (1987).

Robert H. Binstock, The Aged as a Scapegoat, 23 Gerontologist 136-143 (1983).

Daniel Callahan, *Setting Limits: Medical Goals in an Aging Society*, New York: Simon and Schuster, 1987.

James F. Childress, Ensuring Care, Respect, and Fairness for the Elderly, 14 Hastings Center Report 27-31 (Oct. 1984).

Thomas Cole and Sally Gadow, eds., *What Does It Mean to Grow Old? Reflections from the Humanities*, Durham, NC: Duke University Press, 1986.

Steven A. Levenson, Ethical Considerations in Critical and Terminal Illness in the Elderly, 29 Journal of the American Geriatrics Society 563-567 (1981).

Kenneth G. Manton, Changing Concepts of Morbidity and Mortality in the Elderly Population, 60 Milbank Memorial Fund Quarterly 183-244 (1982).

Harry R. Moody, Is It Right to Allocate Health Care Resources on Grounds of Age?, in Elsie L. Bandman and Bertram Bandman, eds., *Bioethics and Human Rights: A Reader for Health Professionals*, Boston: Little, Brown, 1978, pp. 197-201.

Bernice L. Neugarten, *Age or Need? Public Policies for Older People*, Beverly Hills: Sage Publications, 1982.

Francis Pickering, Poverty, Age Discrimination, and Health Care, in George R. Lucas, Jr., ed., *Poverty, Justice, and the Law*, Lanham, MD: University Press of America, 1986, pp. 117-129.

Noralou P. Roos et al., Aging and the Demand for Health Services: Which Aged and Whose Demand?, 24 Gerontologist 31-36 (1984).

Anne A. Scitovsky and Alexander M. Capron, Medical Care at the End of Life: The Interaction of Economics and Ethics, 7 Annual Review of Public Health 59-76 (1986).

Mark Siegler, Should Age be a Criterion in Health Care?, 14 Hastings Center Report 24-27 (Oct. 1984).

David C. Thomasma, Ethical Judgment of Quality of Life in the Care of the Aged, 32 Journal of the American Geriatrics Society 525-527 (1984).

U.S. Congress, Office of Technology Assessment, *Life-Sustaining Technologies and the Elderly*, Washington, DC: U.S. Government Printing Office, 1987.

VI. Accommodating Religious Values and Beliefs

Terrence F. Ackerman, The Limits of Beneficence: Jehovah's Witnesses and Childhood Cancer, 10 Hastings Center Report 13-18 (Aug. 1980).

Jenny Brown, California Penal Code's Child Neglect/Abandonment Statutes: Religious Freedom or Religious Persecution?, 25 Santa Clara Law Review 613-632 (1985).

Paul A. Byrne et al., Brain Death—The Patient, the Physician, and Society, 18 Gonzaga Law Review 429-516 (1982/83).

John Dervin et al., Ethical Considerations in Elder Care, in Mary O'Hara-Devereaux et al., eds., *Elder Care: A Practical Guide to Clinical Geriatrics*, New York: Grune and Stratton, 1981, Ch. 2.

Ruth Faden and Alan Faden, False Belief and the Refusal of Medical Treatment, 3 Journal of Medical Ethics 133-137 (1977).

Sally Gadow, Advocacy Nursing and New Meanings of Aging, 14 Nursing Clinics of North America 81-91 (1979).

David Hilfiker, Allowing the Debilitated to Die:

Facing our Ethical Choices, 308 NEJM 716-719 (1983).

Albert R. Jonsen, Blood Transfusions and Jehovah's Witnesses: The Impact of the Patient's Unusual Beliefs in Critical Care, 2 Critical Care Clinics 91-100 (1986).

Katharine Araujo Miller, Court-Ordered Medical Treatment for Minors: An Alternative Approach to Protect the Child's Best Interests, 7 Whittier Law Review 827-854 (1985).

Lori Leff Mueller, Religious Rights of Children: A Gallery of Judicial Visions, 14 New York University Review of Law and Social Change 323-351 (1986).

New York State Task Force on Life and the Law, *The Determination of Death*, New York, 1986.

Martha Swartz, The Patient Who Refuses Medical Treatment: A Dilemma for Hospitals and Physicians, 11 American Journal of Law and Medicine 147-194 (1985).

LIST OF SELECTED LEGAL AUTHORITIES

This is a list of some of the important cases and other legal authorities relevant to forgoing life-sustaining treatment.

CASES

Barber v. Superior Court, 147 Cal. App. 3d 1006, 195 Cal. Rptr. 484 (Ct. App. 1983).

Bartling v. Superior Court, 163 Cal. App. 3d 186, 209 Cal. Rptr. 220 (Ct. App. 1984), *later appeal, Bartling v. Glendale Adventist Medical Center,* 184 Cal. App. 3d 97, 228 Cal. Rptr. 847 (Ct. App.), *later appeal,* 184 Cal. App. 3d 961, 229 Cal. Rptr. 360 (Ct. App. 1986).

Bouvia v. Superior Court, 179 Cal. App. 3d 1127, 225 Cal. Rptr. 297 (Ct. App.), *review denied* (June 5, 1986).

Brophy v. New England Sinai Hospital, Inc., 398 Mass. 417, 497 N.E.2d 626 (1986).

Canterbury v. Spence, 464 F.2d 772 (D.C. Cir.), *cert. denied,* 409 U.S. 1064 (1972).

In re Colyer, 99 Wash. 2d 114, 660 P.2d 738 (1983).

In re Conroy, 98 N.J. 321, 486 A.2d 1209 (1985).

In re Custody of a Minor, 385 Mass. 697, 434 N.E.2d 601 (1982).

In re Dinnerstein, 6 Mass. App. Ct. 466, 380 N.E.2d 134 (App. Ct. 1978).

In re Eichner (In re Storar), 52 N.Y.2d 363, 420 N.E.2d 64, 438 N.Y.S.2d 266, *cert. denied,* 454 U.S. 858 (1981).

Erickson v. Dilgard, 44 Misc. 2d 27, 252 N.Y.S.2d 705 (1962).

In re Farrell, No. A-76, slip. op. (N.J. June 24, 1987).

In re Guardianship of Hamlin, 102 Wash. 2d 810, 689 P.2d 1372 (1984).

In re Hier, 18 Mass. App. Ct. 200, 464 N.E.2d 959 (App. Ct.), *review denied,* 392 Mass. 1102, 465 N.E.2d 261 (1984).

In re Jobes, No. A-108/109, slip. op. (N.J. June 24, 1987).

John F. Kennedy Memorial Hospital, Inc. v. Bludworth, 452 So. 2d 921 (Fla. 1984).

Leach v. Akron General Medical Center, 68 Ohio Misc. 1, 426 N.E.2d 809 (Com. Pl. 1980), *later proceeding, Estate of Leach v. Shapiro,* 13 Ohio App. 3d 393, 469 N.E.2d 1047 (Ct. App. 1984).

In re L.H.R., 253 Ga. 439, 321 S.E.2d 716 (1984).

In re Lydia E. Hall Hospital, 116 Misc. 2d 477, 455 N.Y.S.2d 706 (Sup. Ct. 1982).

Natanson v. Kline, 186 Kan. 393, 350 P.2d 1093, *clarified,* 187 Kan. 186, 354 P.2d 670 (1960).

People v. Eulo, 63 N.Y.2d 341, 472 N.E.2d 286, 482 N.Y.S.2d 436 (1984).

In re Peter, No. A-78, slip. op. (N.J. June 24, 1987).

In re President and Directors of Georgetown College, Inc., 331 F.2d 1000 (D.C. Cir.), *cert. denied sub nom., Jones v. President and Directors of Georgetown College, Inc.,* 377 U.S. 978 (1964).

In re Quinlan, 70 N.J. 10, 355 A.2d 647, *cert. denied sub nom., Garger v. New Jersey,* 429 U.S. 922 (1976).

Report of the Special January Third Additional 1983 Grand Jury Concerning "Do Not Resuscitate" Procedures at a Certain Hospital in Queens County (Sup. Ct. Queens Co. N.Y. Feb. 8, 1984).

In re Requena, 213 N.J. Super. 443, 517 A.2d 869 (Super. Ct. App. Div. 1986) (per curiam).

Satz v. Perlmutter, 362 So. 2d 160 (Fla. Dist. Ct. App. 1978), *aff'd,* 379 So. 2d 359 (Fla. 1980).

Saunders v. State, 129 Misc. 2d 45, 492 N.Y.S.2d 510 (Sup. Ct. 1985).

Schloendorff v. Society of New York Hospital, 211 N.Y. 125, 105 N.E. 92 (1914).

In re Severns, 425 A.2d 156 (Del. Ch. 1980).

In re Spring, 380 Mass. 629, 405 N.E.2d 115 (1980).

In re Storar, see *In re Eichner* above.

Superintendent of Belchertown State School v. Saikewicz, 373 Mass. 728, 370 N.E.2d 417 (1977).

In re Torres, 357 N.W.2d 332 (Minn. 1984).

In re Visbeck, 210 N.J. Super. 527, 510 A.2d 125 (Super. Ct. Ch. Div. 1986).

In re Maida Yetter, 62 Pa. D. & C.2d 619 (1973).

STATUTES

California Natural Death Act, California Health and Safety Code Ann. Sections 7185-95 (West Supp. 1986).

Child Abuse Amendments of 1984, 42 U.S.C.A. Sections 5101-5103 (West. Supp. 1986).

Uniform Anatomical Gift Act, 8A Uniform Laws Annotated 15-67 (1983).

Uniform Definition of Death Act, 12 Uniform Laws Annotated 270-73 (1986 Supp.).

REGULATIONS

Child Abuse and Neglect Prevention and Treatment, 45 C.F.R. Sections 1340.1-1340.20 (1986).

INDEX

access to health care, 8, 53, 120
  see also equity
acts and omissions, *see* withholding and withdrawing
  treatment
acute care hospitals, 12, 108, 110-17
addiction and pain, 72
admissions to health care settings, 51, 52, 81, 108-17
  see also transfers from health care settings
adequate level of health care, 2, 8, 50, 53, 120, 124, 125
advance directive, 4, 12, 21, 24, 28, 67, 78-84, 109, 110, 113,
  115, 119, 125, 138
  definition of, 78, 140
  revocation of, 81
advance planning, *see* prospective planning
age, as factor in decisionmaking, 33-34, 55, 132-33, 135-37,
  158, 159
antibiotics, iv, 19, 20, 22, 29, 30, 31, 50, 65-68, 82
artificial feeding, *see* nutrition and hydration
assessing patient's ability to understand information, 23,
  39, 40
  see also capacity *and* decisionmaking, capacity of patient
assisting suicide, *see* suicide and assisting suicide
autonomy, *see* self-determination

beneficence, *see* well-being
benefit, 5, 19, 21, 27, 29, 30, 32, 53, 59-60, 61, 65, 66, 73,
  110, 128, 130, 136
  compared to cost, 120-26
  compared to burden, 5-19, 27, 29, 53, 59-60, 61, 65, 66,
    110, 128, 130, 136
best interests standard, 28n
bleeding, treatment for, 19, 20, 22, 29, 30, 31, 34, 46-47,
  52-56, 103, 128
brain death, *see* death, declaration of *and* legislation
burden, 5, 19, 21, 27, 30, 58, 65, 66, 73, 110, 124, 125, 129,
  130, 136
  compared to benefit, 5, 19, 27, 29, 53, 59-60, 61, 65, 66,
    110, 128, 130, 136

capacity, determinations of, 7n, 23, 24, 31, 40, 41, 131-33,
  158
  fluctuating capacity, iv, 22, 27, 133
  uncertain capacity, iv, 22, 27
  see also decisionmaking
cardiac arrest, *see* resuscitation decisions
  cardiopulmonary resuscitation (CPR), definition of, 46,
    140
  see also DNR *and* resuscitation decisions
challenges,
  to assessment of capacity, 23, 31
  to surrogate, 32, 34
  to treatment decision, 32, 34
children, 33-34, 55, 98
comatose patients, *see* irreversibly unconscious patients

comfort, *see* palliative care
communication,
  between patient and responsible health care profes-
    sional, 9-12, 18-22, 27, 31, 38, 39, 40, 47-50, 51, 53,
    61, 62, 66-67, 78, 80, 81, 109, 110, 123
  between surrogate and responsible health care profes-
    sional, 10, 19, 22, 31, 38, 40, 47-50, 51, 53, 61, 62, 66-
    67, 103, 110
  within health care team, 20-21, 23, 31, 32, 39, 41, 50, 54,
    62
  see also informed consent *and* surrogate, decisionmaking
competence, 7n, 131-32
  see also capacity *and* decisionmaking
cost containment, 120, 124, 158
  see also economic considerations
costs of care, 8, 27, 42, 75, 119, 120
  see also economic considerations
costworthy care, 51, 115, 120-26, 158
  see also economic considerations
court review, *see* judicial review
CPR, *see* DNR *and* resuscitation decisions
criminal law, 3, 4, 129
  intentional killing, 6, 73, 128-29, 130-31
  see also law, role of

death, 86-98, 138
  declaration of, 86, 91-92, 159
  intended vs. unintended but foreseeable, 73, 128-29, 130-
    31
decisionmaking, iv, 2-9, 13, 18-34, 38, 46, 47, 48, 50, 65, 66,
  131-33, 135-37
  by patients with capacity, iv, 7, 19, 22, 26-28, 39, 40, 41,
    48-50, 74, 75, 78, 80, 128, 131, 134, 137
  by patients with fluctuating capacity or uncertain capac-
    ity, iv, 22, 27
  by patients without capacity, iv, 7, 19, 22-27, 33, 34, 48-
    50, 54, 67, 74, 78, 80, 82, 128, 131, 134
  capacity of patient, 7, 23, 24, 40, 74, 82, 131-33, 158
  changing decisions, 31, 133
  competence and incompetence, 7, 131-32
  in hospices, 12, 108
  in hospitals, 12, 49, 108, 110, 111
  in nursing homes, 12, 49, 108, 114-16
  review of, 25-26, 31-32, 34, 50, 51, 62, 74, 81, 105, 110,
    113
  role of family in, iii, 18, 22, 23, 54, 81, 89, 137, 158
  role of friends in, 12, 22, 23, 81, 88
  see also communication *and* surrogate
dialysis, iii, 4, 20, 22, 27, 38, 39, 41, 42, 50
disabling condition, 28-29, 49, 134, 158
disagreement, 13, 20, 23, 31-33, 34, 50, 66, 68, 100, 104-
  105, 158-59
  among family and friends, 23
  between patient or surrogate and responsible health care
    professional, 20, 31-33, 34, 50, 66, 68, 100, 104-105,
    158-59
  within health care team, 31, 32, 33

154

resuscitation decisions, iv, 4, 20, 22, 30, 31, 34, 46-52, 82, 112, 158
    and adequate level of care, 49, 50, 112
    and competent patients, 47
    costs of, 52
    definition of, 140
    delay in, 51
    orders against, 29, 46, 47, 50
    presumption favoring, 49, 51
    see also DNR
right to privacy, *see* privacy

sanctity of life, 9
sedation, *see* pain medication
self-determination, 2, 7, 8, 10, 19, 51, 73, 120, 121, 125, 128-33, 137, 138
    affected by institutions, 114, 129
    well-being in conflict with, 53
stress, 31, 49, 50, 54, 67
substituted judgment standard, 28n
suffering, 6, 27, 28, 60, 71, 73
    see also palliative care *and* pain, accompanying the dying process
suicide and assisting suicide, vs. refusal of treatment, 6, 73, 128-29, 158
supportive care, 30, 40, 42, 59, 61, 67, 71, 75
    see also palliative care
surrogate, iii, iv, 83, 88, 103, 114, 158
    decisionmaking, 7, 10, 11, 19, 22-24, 27, 28, 32, 47, 50, 66, 67, 73, 74, 80-84, 128, 134-36, 158
    definition of, 141
    family member as, 18, 23, 81, 158
    friend as, 23, 81
    identification of, 23-26, 110
    multiple, 23
    patients who lack, 11, 24-26, 158
    see also challenges, to surrogate
surrogates committee, 25
symptom control, *see* palliative care

terminally ill (patients), 28, 49, 65
    definition of, iii, 141
    symptoms in, 71
termination of life-sustaining treatment, iv, 2-11, 19, 28-31, 41, 46, 47, 50-55, 59, 61, 73, 89, 109-12, 116, 128-30, 133, 137, 158
    see also withholding and withdrawing treatment
therapy, failure to initiate vs. stopping, *see* withholding and withdrawing treatment
time-limited trial of intervention, 30, 50, 60, 61, 130
transfers from health care settings, 32, 33, 51, 83, 108-17
    see also admissions to health care settings
transfusion, *see* bleeding, treatment for
transplantation, *see* organ transplantation
treatment directive, 28, 78, 79, 81, 82
    definition of, 80, 141
    see also advance directive *and* proxy directive

treatment refusal, *see* decisionmaking *and* withholding and withdrawing treatment

unconscious (patients), *see* irreversibly unconscious patients
Uniform Determination of Death Act, *see* death, declaration of
    see also legislation

ventilators, iv, 4, 20, 22, 24, 27, 30, 34, 38-41, 50
    weaning from, 39, 41
voluntariness of decision to forgo life-sustaining treatment, 54

well-being, iii, iv, 7, 19, 66, 73, 120, 123, 125, 131, 132, 158
withholding and withdrawing treatment, 5, 6, 19, 29, 30, 38, 130-31
wrongful death, *see* criminal law

APPENDIX: Dissents

The following dissents to specific Sections of the Guidelines have been submitted by members of the project group. The project director and associate directors do not necessarily agree that these dissents in each instance accurately depict the positions actually taken in the Guidelines. Readers should refer to the specific Sections cited to make that determination for themselves.

Dissent of Leslie Steven Rothenberg

The ethical distinction between "terminating treatment" and "terminating life" (whether called active euthanasia, mercy killing, assisted suicide, or "medical killing") may be more important to me than to others, particularly because the health care system is preoccupied with cost containment and because society undervalues persons with disabilities (including those that accompany advanced age). For all these reasons, I dissent from the following sections of this report:

1. **PART ONE:** Section (4) (c) 3, pp. 28-29: I dissent from including patients with a "disabling condition that is severe and irreversible" and those with "irreversible loss of consciousness" in the patient categories for whom terminating treatment is said to be especially appropriate.

2. **PART TWO:** Section B (2) (b), p. 49; I dissent from the language that singles out patients with a "disabling condition that is severe and irreversible" and patients who have "suffered an irreversible loss of consciousness" as persons whose views (or whose surrogate's views) on cardiopulmonary resuscitation (CPR) should be discussed.

3. **PART TWO:** Section C, p. 57: I dissent from the entirety of this Section except as it pertains to patients whose death is expected within a few days, or for whom nutrition cannot be provided successfully because they have lost the ability to metabolize.

4. **INTRODUCTION,** Section II, p. 6 and **PART SIX:** Section I, p. 128: I dissent because they do not take a stronger stand against active euthanasia and assisting suicide.

I fear these Guidelines, if widely endorsed, may be used to give a moral "imprimatur" to undertreating or failing to treat persons with disabilities, unconscious persons for whom accurate prognoses are not yet obtainable, elderly patients with severe dementia, and others whose treatment is not believed (to use the language from PART FIVE: Section C, p. 118, etc.) "costworthy."

Dissent of Robert M. Veatch

Determining Capacity and the Surrogate Process

Responsible health care professionals have no legal or moral authority to determine decision-making capacity (*cf.* PART ONE: Section (3) (a), p. 23). Unless the patient, family, and responsible health care professional agree that the patient lacks capacity, or the patient is silent when asked, the patient must be presumed to have capacity. Only courts may use a process standard in determining capacity; others must use a status standard (*cf.* PART SIX: Section III, p. 131). Next-of-kin must act as a surrogate until a court directs otherwise; permitting others to act as surrogates violates state law and patient rights. Responsible health care professionals should never choose the surrogate (*cf.* PART ONE: Section (3) (b), p. 24). Patients without surrogates should have them court-appointed, unless the patient falls into a category publicly authorized for nontreatment. Bonded surrogates (*i.e.,* those who are not strangers to the patient) must have discretion to choose among reasonable treatment options or familial autonomy would be violated and constant judicial intervention would be required (*cf.* PART ONE: Section (3) (c), p. 26). Only stranger guardians must follow the single most reasonable course.

Institutional Ethics Committees (IECs)

IEC referral can be valuable, as long as the patient/surrogate approves. However, the patient/surrogate may prefer another moral advisor, and consulting IECs without patient/surrogate consent always violates confidentiality (*cf.* PART ONE: Sections (8), p. 31; PART FIVE: Sections A, II (5), p. 102 and (9) (c), p. 104). Normally patients/surrogates should participate in IEC proceedings, but some may prefer other advisors to participate in their stead (*cf.* PART FIVE: Section A, II (9) (f), p. 104). IECs should never deal with resource allocation ethics, because this conflicts with IECs' ethical duty to serve patients (*cf.* PART FIVE: Section A, II (9) (d), p. 104).

Economic Considerations

National and local policies must place moral limits on low-priority benefits as well as useless or harmful care. The criterion should never be maximizing utility (benefit/cost), but the rights of the worst off patients (*cf.* PART FIVE: Section C, I, p. 119).

Judgments should be based on well-being over a lifetime. Older persons have had society's resources over more years, so in some cases chronological age (rather than physiological) is a just allocation basis (*cf.* PART FIVE: Section C, I p. 119; PART SIX: Section V, p. 135).

Defining Death

Defining death is a policy matter that ought to be resolved by statute or judicial process. Physician use of unauthorized definitions of death is wrong (*cf.* PART FOUR: Section I, p. 87). Institutional policy or legal counsel cannot authorize other definitions (*cf.* PART FOUR: Section II (2), p. 88).

States should now adopt a definition of death which provides that the irrevocable loss of higher brain functions constitutes death unless the patient/surrogate opts for a whole brain or cardio-respiratory definition (*cf.* PART FOUR: Section I, p. 86). The claim that allowing individual options creates intolerable "confusion" is implausible (*cf.* PART SIX: Section VI, p. 138). The law can handle health and life insurance problems, etc. (*e.g.,* Medicare coverage could cease for living brain dead persons). Moreover, respecting treatment refusal choices has greater impact on insurance and no one fears "confusion." The rights of religious and other minorities are vital and cannot be avoided by authorizing the treatment of corpses.